Life Without Obesity

Lose weight without starving or counting calories.

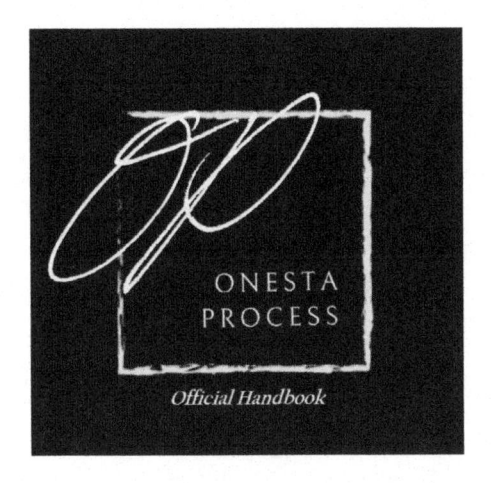

ONESTA PROCESS

Official Handbook

Joseph A. Onesta

www.josephonesta.com

www.mindpowerpittsburgh.com

Life Without Obesity

Lose weight without starving or counting calories.

Copyright © 2022 by Joseph A. Onesta

All rights reserved. No part of this publication may be reproduced, stored in a retrieval system, reproduced, distributed, or transmitted in any form or by any means, including photocopying, recording, or other electronic or mechanical methods, without the prior written permission of the author, except in the case of brief quotations embodied in critical reviews and certain other non-commercial uses permitted by copyright law.

ISBN: 979-8-9872548-1-3

Integrity HPI

Human Performance Improvement

To contact the author, visit: www.mindpowerpittsburgh.com or www.josephonesta.com.

Certain content and portions of this book have been previously published under the titles *The Hypnofasting Program Guide* (2020), *Deleting Diabetes* (2022), *Life Without Diabetes,* (2022), and *The Hypnotist's Guide to Diabetes and Obesity* (2022)

This book is dedicated to everyone who has chosen to take ownership and responsibility for their own wellness. A special thanks to the clients who, along the way, shared their experiences, their feelings, and occasionally, their frustrations.

Table of Contents

Chapter One: Who the Hell Am I?....................1

Chapter Two: Stop Blaming Yourself....................7

Chapter Three: How We Get Fat....................17

Chapter Four: Toward a New Normal....................35

Chapter Five: Stage One....................51

Chapter Six: Hunger, Cravings, and Emotional Eating...61

Chapter Seven: Stage Two....................77

Chapter Eight: Food....................87

Chapter Nine: Stage Three....................103

Chapter Ten: Checking in....................117

Chapter Eleven: Stage Four....................127

Chapter Twelve: Opposition, Ketosis, and Autophagy.137

Chapter Thirteen: Stage Five....................152

Chapter Fourteen: Genetics and Metabolism....................161

Chapter Fifteen: The Home Stretch....................173

Recommended Reading....................177

About the Author....................179

Chapter One: Who the Hell Am I?

Let's let that elephant roam the room freely. I am not a doctor. I'm not a nutritionist. I'm not a scientist. Neither am I an idiot. I get that I lack the credentials to construct a weight loss program and even to write a book such as this. However, I am a formerly obese person who was and is no longer a Type 2 diabetic. At the time of writing this book, I am 61 years old. I am about 100 pounds lighter than I was. Apart from a pound or two in either direction, I've remained the same for four years.

When I began my journey in my late 50s, I had given up hope of losing any amount of weight. I weighed 300 pounds, give or take a few. I was well experienced at dieting. For different stretches of time, I have either maintained or given up on strenuous exercise programs. It didn't seem to matter what I did, the results were temporary.

So nearly four years ago, my doctor wanted to put me on a third diabetes medication just prior to prescribing injectable insulin. My A1c (a three-month average of blood sugar levels) was through the roof, despite my faithfully taking my medications and adhering to the dietary advice I had been given. The progression of the disease scared me, and I decided to look for alternatives.

I found lots of them, but only one that made any scientific sense. I've never met anyone who substantially benefited from the supplements touted to control blood sugar. But discovering the low-carb and intermittent fasting communities, I met people who could demonstrate the benefits they received even if the things they did seemed somewhat extreme. Who, after all, wants to fast or cut down on carbs? However, these folks, many of them physicians, cited sound scientific studies which back up their claims.

I made some mistakes along the way. I tried a lot of different things and in the end, I created what is now called The Onesta Process™. This is a combination of several strategies that, when applied gradually and with some compromise on an individual level, guide followers into a comfortable and sustainable lifestyle.

As I said, I had given up entirely on permanent weight loss but my investigations into the functions of the body, the organs, and the digestive system as well as the role of nutrients and the benefits of temporary fasting not only allowed my body to heal the diabetes, I lost a ton of weight.

My clinical hypnosis office was located in a wellness center. I remember the day one of the massage therapists came up to me and congratulated me on my weight loss while chastising me for my slovenly appearance. "You are a professional and you need to dress like one. You need to go shopping."

I must have known I was losing weight because I had to drill several new holes in my belt. But I was so focused on my blood sugar levels that I just didn't pay attention. Anyone with excess fat around the middle knows that one can always tighten the belt to bite into the layers of fat. I just kept tightening my belt.

Honestly, I can admit now that there must have been some body dysmorphia, as if I were simply imagining that I was still as fat as I had been. I didn't see the weight coming off despite the baggy clothes and the extra holes in my belt. I had been fat for so long that I still saw myself as fat, despite discovering that I had lost more than 10 inches off my waist.

Today, my waist size is the same as it was the day I graduated from high school, 34 inches, though I prefer a size 36 when having to cope with skinnier cuts. Of course, my body isn't the same. My skin isn't as tight, especially after losing all that weight. I don't exactly carry my weight the way I did at 17.

I graduated from high school in 1978. Most of the boys my age back then wore size 28 or 30 inches. At 34 inches, I was considered fat. Today, finding a 17- or 18-year-old boy with a waist size of 28 inches is rare and he might be considered on the skinny side of thin. In the intervening years, the average waist circumference for men has increased considerably. A boy graduating high school with a waist size of 34 inches would today be seen as ideal. We've grown fatter, obesity is far more common, and Type 2 diabetes is increasingly common even among children.

I know what it means and how it feels to be obese. I don't shy away from using the word obese, although I have felt the very real sting of having it applied to me. Given the title of this book, I imagine you are standing up to the word as well. Congratulations. It takes immense personal strength to come to terms with such a negative label. We know the feeling of hopelessness associated with repeated attempts to lose weight. We share the history of self-blame we heap on our shoulders for being unable to achieve or sustain our weight loss goals. We know the feelings of anger, self-hate, cursed weakness, unavoidable guilt, and inherent frustration that weight loss and fat-shaming encompass.

In the following pages, I'm going to introduce you to the science behind obesity in a way that just about anyone can understand. I will not demand that you read scientific studies. I won't even present them to you. This book contains a recommended reading list and if you are truly interested in the science behind the claims made in this book, I direct you to the physicians and investigative reporters who have thoroughly explored the science.

The hardest part of learning what I had to learn and what I will share with you is coming to terms with and acknowledging that what we have been taught by the diet and exercise industry—and what was reaffirmed by much of the medical and nutritional professions—has been misguided, based on assumptions rather than science. It is, for lack of a more precise word, simply wrong.

Before we begin, allow me to promise that if you follow my process:

- You will not starve. You may feel a bit of hunger at the beginning of the process but we're used to that and I promise it won't last.
- You will likely need to eat more than you currently do.
- You will understand what is going on in your body and your trust in your body will increase.
- Your body will change.
- Your tastes will change.
- We will not count calories, points, units, carbs, or anything else.
- Your whole relationship with food will change.
- Changes are gradual, natural, and comfortable.
- You will feel better.
- You will be healthier.

- You will have more energy.
- You will be more alert.
- Your life will be happier and you will feel more in control.
- Best of all, this will be the last time you readdress the life-long plague of weight loss struggles. What we will do in this process is establish a new normal in your life.

Are you ready? Let's go, then.

Chapter Two: Stop Blaming Yourself

"I used to step on the scale each morning and then beat myself up for the rest of the day." — Stephanie D.

In my clinical hypnosis practice, I meet a lot of people who blame themselves for the situations in which they find themselves. They come to see me to make changes in how they think, react, and in what they do.

I have the distinct pleasure of advising you that you are not to blame for your weight problem. It's not your fault. You've been gaslighted. You've been told either directly or indirectly that you are fat because you are a lazy glutton who eats too much and doesn't exercise enough. You've been told that weight control is calorie control and that if you exercise you burn calories. That's total bullshit! Sorry about my language but I can't think of a better term, right now. You likely believe that you can cut calories by replacing meals with vitamin-enriched milkshakes, protein bars, low-fat products, and by using artificial sweeteners, like those found in diet sodas. You've been taught that a healthy diet is firmly based on whole grain products like bread, pasta, and cereals. You have been persuaded that manufactured and processed foods are healthy because they are vitamin enriched. I may have shocked you but by the time we are done with this process, a very new you will be convinced of the truth of these statements, and much, if not all of that bullshit will be mucked out.

Unless you are as old as I am, you might not remember anyone telling you that a snack would "spoil your dinner." That thought went out of vogue in the early 1970s. By then, stay-at-home mothers were becoming increasingly rare, latch-key kids more common, and home-cooked meals were sometimes replaced with takeout food and frozen entrees known as TV dinners. Easy-to-prepare processed or packaged foods like chicken nuggets, fish sticks, and mac and cheese began to fill our freezers and shelves.

Perhaps it was the ready-to-eat nature of these processed foods that gradually became grazing fodder. Kids come home and pop pizza rolls, fries, or popcorn into the microwave to tide them over until dinner, whereas before kids were told to wait. When my mother warned me not to spoil my dinner, dinner time was two or three hours later. A gap of two or three hours without nibbling may seem inconceivable to many people today. Three square meals a day is a thing of the past.

Drive-through windows provided supersized combo selections on the go so that as a culture, we no longer thought in terms of meals but convenient servings on the run and we rarely realized how much or how often we consumed processed food products. Anyone who has ever worked in a restaurant can attest that the vast majority of the food comes frozen, prepared, ready to heat, sell, and eat.

Of course, manufacturers of processed food wanted to make their food as marketable and delicious as possible because it would mean more sales and a bigger share of the market. Old-fashioned TV dinners, something one had to experience to understand the true degree of disappointment, were replaced with tastier, often microwaveable food products that resemble things we might have made at home. Processed food manufacturers perfected a thing called the *bliss bite*, a combination of fat, salt, and sugar that would be delicious and ever-so-slightly addictive.

At the same time, a cultural food war was raging over the potential dietary cause of heart disease. A man named Ancel Keys championed the idea that saturated fat (fat from animal sources) clogged arteries with cholesterol. The scientific validity of his conclusions was justifiably challenged at the time, but his charisma and persuasive abilities won the day. Out went fat, and in came polyunsaturated seed oils, more sugar, sugar derivatives, and chemically produced flavor enhancers.

In full complicity with Keys' theories, in 1980, the food and drug administration began promoting the food pyramid. The base of that pyramid consisted of grains and cereals—in other words, carbohydrates—most of which were highly processed and refined to the point that if they were to offer any nutritional value at all, vitamins would have to be added to the recipe. Processing removes the fiber, making the texture and flavor more appealing, and the manufacturing process easier to control.

Because of the supposedly unhealthy nature of saturated fat, carbohydrates took center stage in our meal planning and restaurant menus, replacing meat (especially red meat) with smaller and leaner cuts of meat. We now fill our plates with starches; potatoes and pasta abound. As we embraced these changes, even our language changed. We used to say, "meat and vegetables," but now one more commonly hears "fruits and vegetables," placing fruit on par with vegetables. Fruit in many cultures is justifiably considered a desert, not a vegetable, despite being found in the same section of the supermarket.

At one point there was an absolute kerfuffle over the healthiness of eggs, as evidenced by two conflicting covers of *Time* magazine. The issues at hand weighed the value of the protein eggs provided against the cholesterol found in the yolks. Despite the evidence that removing saturated fat from our diets did nothing to improve cardiovascular health, many doctors and nutritionists continued to warn their patients against saturated fat and continued recommending a diet based on grains as the healthy choice.

Ironically, it is the proliferation of carbohydrates in our diet that pose the greatest dietary risk to cardiovascular health. Cardiovascular risk is a factor of metabolic disease which we now understand is a function of excess carbohydrates in the diet which raises blood glucose and triggers elevated levels of insulin. Did I just make you dizzy? Trust me. You'll understand every word before we are through.

The same thing happened with milk and dairy products. Since animal fat was considered bad, taking the fat out of milk seemed like a good idea, until no one knew what to do with all that milk fat. The first answer was cheese, of course. Cheese was soon highly promoted and available in all sorts of easy-to-use processed forms. But the next horrifying step was soon to follow. Low-fat or non-fat cheese made its rubbery way into our lives because heart disease continued to rise, and where were we getting that bad fat? It had to be the cheese. Processors had to find a way of making something taste like cheese without being cheese. Hydrogenated vegetable oils, now known as trans fats, replaced saturated fat, and cheese was no longer cheese. Now we have a thing called "cheese food," which is actually less than 50% cheese. Read the ingredients to find out what replaced the missing 51% that used to be cheese, if you dare.

I point out that as an extension of Keys' theories and

the broad acceptance of their validity despite sound evidence to the contrary, these shifts were both accepted and propagated by the medical and nutrition professions. In many cases, they are still. Once accepted, the theory proposed by Ancel Keys became a veritably unassailable dogma. Professionals who opposed his position were disregarded and maligned. Despite the fact that parallel to these changes, cardiovascular disease as well as many other conditions now associated with metabolic disease, such as obesity and Type 2 diabetes, actually *increased*.

However, instead of looking back on the changes we had made as the potential source of the growing problem, researchers looked for ways of addressing what they saw as emerging *new* problems. Medications to lower blood pressure, lower cholesterol levels, and control blood glucose levels were the preferred solutions.

It is unfortunate that the majority of the parties involved in the spread of misinformation either remain unaware of their error or cannot simply admit that they were wrong. The scientists, government officials, medical and insurance systems, doctors, and nutritionists who still promote procedures based on Keys' theory resist change and find it difficult to consider the conflicting evidence.

In the end, we need to educate ourselves. When our doctors make a recommendation, we need to understand that it may be based on the most up-to-date science, but then again it might be based on something one of their professors said in med school. We also have to add the fact that much of the advice of our doctors is dictated by standard procedures from diagnostic protocols to which medications can or cannot be prescribed. Very little of what a general practitioner might consider is the mind-body relationship, at least not until the doctor runs out of options.

When doctors tell you that you need to lose weight, how do you feel? Do your doctors truly understand what you have gone through? Do they even ask you about it or do you feel like they don't believe you have been trying? Do *you* believe you have been trying or do you even doubt your own efforts?

I hope you can now see that you and I are just two of many who have been influenced and persuaded into believing something that simply isn't true, that the metabolic model we follow is flawed. I honestly do not believe that Ancel Keys intended any harm. I think he wanted to help. His assertions seemed logical and his charisma won the day. Like others in history, he likely wanted to make a name for himself, though I doubt he would have really wanted his growing negative reputation. He probably wanted to be a hero and convinced himself, despite the intentional flaws in his research, that he was doing the right thing.

His theories resulted in a veritable gold rush for food manufacturers, fueled the growth of industrial agriculture, and was likely the impetus behind the genetic modification of vegetables to increase production and shelf-life. It really looks like a big conspiracy to make us fat and dependent on pharmaceuticals. Although I doubt that any kind of real conspiracy existed. I think they were all well-intentioned. However, I have no doubt that some people, recognizing the trend, most likely took advantage and profited from it.

You and I and countless others who have together contributed to the rising statistics of corpulence and associated health problems are victims of circumstance. It was unfair. It was wrong. We are paying the price but it is not our fault. We bought into the growing lie because we believed without question what we were told. We did what we thought was the right thing to do. Without having to place blame on others, we can throw off that same blame from our own shoulders and actually *do* something to fix the problem in our lives and in our society.

Getting angry about this problem only helps if it motivates you to change your own experience. I was fearful and sought answers. When I found them, I became angry. But, as a hypnotist, I understand that stagnant anger breeds bitterness, and bitterness creates an environment of hopelessness. I changed my experience and now I am passionate about helping as many people as I can to lose as much weight and reverse metabolic disease as they can.

My own doctor's reaction to my change has been nothing short of skeptical and suspicious. "The numbers don't lie," was his only concession. I am sure he didn't expect it to last. After three years, he finally asked me what hypnosis had to do with my change. I explained to him that no one wants to do what we have to do. No one thinks they can do it until they do it. That is where hypnosis comes in. You *can* do it. Hypnosis, whether self-hypnosis or working with a qualified professional, will make it easier. But you still have to do it.

In this book, I'll provide you with mind hacks, a kind of self-hypnosis technique that will help you do it on your own. If you struggle with it (and some of you will), I urge you to not give up but find a hypnotist trained in the Onesta Process. We are out there. If we aren't physically close to you, most of us work online.

For now, however, just take a moment and make a decision to be willing to help yourself. Understand that you need to unlearn some old things, learn some new things, and allow your mind to change. Back in my days in the ministry, I loved this verse in the bible that reads, "Do not conform to the patterns of this world but be transformed by the renewing of your mind." (Romans 12:2, NIV) I think it is very apt for this context.

You have to give up worrying about calories. You have to eat enough for your body to understand that you are not starving. Therefore, you must not starve yourself. You have to learn about how your body works, how it processes what you eat and what criteria to use to choose food that will best benefit your body. The best part is that when you feed your body good, wholesome food, the things you **want** to eat change.

In the Onesta process, you will always be in charge of the

choices you make. It is my job to educate and advise you of the nature of those choices and to help you understand which choices are better than others. You choose. You decide. You act.

In my clinical practice, I have found that every client requires one form of compromise or another so the Onesta Process is not written in stone. Most of the compromises are temporary while the mind is changing. Changes you might find difficult to accept today may be nothing to you in a few weeks. Just be willing to be willing. Take it one step or stage at a time and you will find the right balance that fits your life.

I'd like to end this chapter with a mind-hack. So often, in terms of losing weight, we use the phrase, "I can't." From this point forward, when that phrase or feeling comes to mind, simply change it to, "I feel like I can't right now, but I can—right now."

Chapter Three: How We Get Fat

Take the Quiz.

Answer true or false to the following questions then tally your answers.

1. People who are overweight lack willpower.
2. People who are overweight need to exercise more.
3. People who are overweight eat too much.
4. In order to exercise properly, you have to sweat and your heart rate must increase.
5. Proper exercise should happen at least three times a week for at least 30 minutes.
6. It is better to eat smaller snacks multiple times a day rather than three full meals.
7. Obesity causes heart disease.
8. Obesity causes diabetes.

9. Obesity is genetically determined.
10. We should eat when we feel hungry.
11. The key to losing weight is to eat less and exercise more.
12. We exercise to burn calories.
13. All calories are equal; a calorie is a calorie.
14. Obesity reflects the character of the person.
15. Cravings are impossible to resist.
16. Feelings of hunger are biological.
17. Carbohydrates are a necessary element of a healthy diet.
18. A plant-based diet is healthier than one that includes meat.

The above statements are all false. How did you do?

In this chapter, we will explore metabolic science, but I won't bore you with a bunch of data. Most people would fall asleep reading through articles reporting scientific studies. My presentation is a summary of the ever-growing body of metabolic science. I won't cite studies directly, however; it has been done in more detail than I have room for here.

If you are science-minded and want to dig your teeth into that material, the best place to start is the recommended reading list at the end of this book. Writing for the general public in easy-to-understand ways, those authors are qualified physicians and investigative reporters who present material filled with citations that will help you find the original sources. As for me, I will just stick to the easy-to-read style.

Our bodies need energy and nutrition. Nutrition keeps the gears greased and energy keeps the engine running.

Glucose is the primary fuel of the body. The easiest and fastest sources of glucose are carbohydrates such as sugar, grains, and starchy vegetables. But these are not the only sources of glucose. Some of the protein you consume is converted into glucose and your body is capable of producing glucose on its own.

If you are overweight, you have some degree of insulin resistance. Insulin resistance happens when there is too much glucose in the blood and the cells of the body already have all the glucose they can handle. When body cells are full, they begin pushing push away from the glucose table. They resist taking on more glucose.

Excess glucose cannot remain in the bloodstream without serious consequences. It just can't keep circulating in the blood until it is needed. The body has places to store excess glucose. Insulin is the hormone that directs glucose to places of storage.

If there is excess glucose, the pancreas will create more insulin in an attempt to force the glucose into cells. Chronically high levels of insulin due to consistent excess glucose is a condition called *hyperinsulinemia*. When the cells become increasingly resistant, insulin directs the excess glucose to the liver where it is converted to a limited amount of glycogen and an unlimited amount of fat.

When blood glucose levels drop below normal, the liver will take the glycogen and easily convert it back into glucose so that the cells have a ready supply. What happens if we continue eating glucose-generating food? More and more excess glucose is funneled into the liver. The liver never really has much of a chance to use glycogen so virtually all of that excess glucose is directed toward long-term storage as fat, first around the organs and then all around the body. Fat is simply stored energy.

If you are overweight but not yet diabetic, you now understand what is happening. All carbohydrates (including complex ones) are converted into glucose. This is why people who go on a ketogenic diet initially lose weight, a subject we will explore at length later. Reducing carbohydrate intake sufficiently to no longer create excess glucose stops the process of creating fat and allows the body to actually use fat as a fuel source. If you simply do a ketogenic diet for a while, you will lose weight. But just like any other diet, once you stop, you'll easily regain weight. If you go back to doing what you did before, you go back to being the way you were before.

You may also now begin to understand how Type 2 diabetes develops. Continued consumption of food that is readily converted into glucose fatigues the pancreas. Eventually, it will not be able to produce enough insulin to sufficiently remove the glucose from the blood. Blood sugar levels begin to rise, and the doctor begins talking about diabetes. Medications will be prescribed to help the pancreas do its job. However, the treatment of blood glucose levels does not address the *cause* of the problem, which is excess glucose demanding excess insulin. Directly treating blood glucose levels is important but can only help temporarily. The cause of the problem, excess glucose and hyperinsulinemia, are still present and getting worse.

Carbohydrates have the most dramatic elevating effect on blood glucose. Proteins, such as meat, fish, poultry, eggs, and dairy have a moderate effect on blood glucose levels. Dietary fat, though vilified for decades because of its calorie content and the reputation it gained under the theories of Ancel Keys, has very little effect on blood glucose and thus does not contribute to obesity. Let me repeat, **consuming dietary fat does not contribute to obesity**. Surprise! It thus stands to reason that reducing carbohydrates delivers the best results and explains the epidemic levels of obesity that resulted after we began following the food pyramid back in the 1980s.

It seems that insulin resistance and hyperinsulinemia have a chicken-and-egg relationship. They form a kind of cycle that feeds into one another over time. Insulin resistance demands more insulin to direct blood glucose and increased insulin develops insulin resistance. In the simplest way of understanding it, if we continually stimulate increasing amounts of insulin, insulin resistance will develop. Insulin resistance leads to weight gain and other symptomatic conditions of metabolic disease.

If only there were a way of testing for hyperinsulinemia! If there were, we'd know we were consuming too many carbohydrates and we could avoid getting fat in the first place.

Actually, there is. It's called a fasting insulin test, and it can be part of a regular metabolic panel screening. Why the test is not routine is a matter of conjecture. One suggestion might be that allopathic medicine has nothing to prescribe for elevated insulin levels. There are no medications for it because they could prove fatal. Lowering insulin would raise blood glucose to dangerous levels. The core answer to the problem is reducing the need for excess insulin.

Another, perhaps more obvious reason why fasting insulin is not measured is that there are no early signs of hyperinsulinemia. The pancreas is working harder than it should and is doing a good job of it. A doctor might not test for metabolic disease until there are obvious signs such as increasing weight or rising blood pressure.

When I first was diagnosed with Type 2 diabetes, the doctor told me I could control the progression of the disease with diet, exercise, and a pill. He did not explain the diet in detail but sent me to a nutritionist. He gave me a prescription for metformin and told me to lose weight and get more exercise.

I had been hearing the admonition to lose weight and exercise more for years. After countless attempts at altering my diet and thousands of wasted dollars on gym memberships, all my efforts to lose weight and keep it off were disappointing. After a while, I learned to live with being fat and accepted feeling helpless and guilty for it.

The nutritionist's advice was the standard offered at the

time: I should get about 60% of my calories from complex carbohydrates and eat more frequent, smaller meals every two hours or so to keep my blood sugar levels stable.

As far as maintaining blood glucose levels, the advice was good but in the long term, it was wrong. It did nothing to address hyperinsulinemia, which is arguably the root condition of metabolic disease. You'll come to understand that the advice I received was precisely the opposite of what needs to be done if one wishes to reverse Type 2 diabetes.

Here's a simplified explanation of how it works. We eat. The food is digested. Depending on what we have eaten, micronutrients like vitamins and proteins are extracted and fuel (usually glucose) is created. Under the supervision of insulin, glucose is distributed to every cell in the body to be used as fuel to perform cellular functions. Extra glucose is then funneled into the liver. The liver converts the glucose into glycogen, keeping about a day's worth of reserves to be used when the body requires it. If there is still extra glucose, the liver stashes it into fat reserves. Ironically, fat cells are rarely insulin resistant.

Blood glucose usually hits a high point after eating and then begins to drop. Again, depending on what we've eaten, that spike might be dramatic or mild, and the drop may be slow or precipitous. (That feeling of sleepiness after eating a sweet meal like Thanksgiving dinner is only partly the tryptophan in the turkey. It's mostly a precipitous drop in blood glucose.)

The longer we go without eating, the body begins to regulate the level of blood glucose by accessing the glycogen stores in the liver and converting it back into glucose. It is also using tiny amounts of fat in this process, because the body needs fat to function properly. If the liver's glycogen stores become depleted, it begins to dip into the fat stores in a greater way, converting fat first into glucose and then into ketones.

If we don't eat for significantly longer or we greatly restrict our caloric intake, the body can go into a kind of starvation or semi-starvation mode that often includes two facets. One that people see in a positive light is autophagy, which means the body increases its use of old cells as fuel. Under extreme conditions, this process can be viewed as a *wasting* condition. If you've ever seen someone diminished by a long-term illness, or you've seen photos of Nazi death camp survivors, you see the emaciation caused by extreme starvation and autophagy.

The other aspect is a slowing down of metabolism and a more conservative use of energy in order to sustain life itself. This slowed metabolic rate is another reason why it is so easy to regain weight after stopping or easing up on a diet.

The Onesta Process is not a diet but a shift in lifestyle. Many of the changes you embrace will become part of your new lifestyle. Most of what we will do isn't temporary.

Metabolic syndrome is the result of a lifestyle that demands increasing amounts of insulin to do the job of getting glucose out of the blood and into the cells. The eventual inability of the pancreas to produce enough insulin has two possible causes. The pancreas could be damaged in some way but the more likely scenario is that the individual has habitually consumed foods that elevate blood glucose levels. For years, the pancreas has been doing an outstanding job of managing mounting blood glucose. As the barrage continues, insulin resistance increases, and symptomatic conditions begin to appear. Again, the most common early arrivals are obesity and high blood pressure. The pancreas reaches maximum insulin production, blood sugar levels begin to climb, and a diagnosis of other symptomatic conditions such as fatty liver, prediabetes, or Type 2 diabetes results.

The process can be reversed. In this case, your body will respond positively and begin healing. We can do it quickly or in a paced manner. The more quickly we work, the more dramatic the results. However, those results may be less sustainable because while the behaviors have changed *temporarily*, the mindset remains the same. Synchronizing mind changes with body changes often takes time. The unconscious mind doesn't trust rapid changes. It doesn't see them as changes but rather as temporary conditions with which it must cope.

People who have bariatric surgery, for example, often experience a rapid but temporary reversal of Type 2 diabetes. Upwards of 60% of those who have bariatric surgery regain the weight despite the changes that have been made to their digestive system. Unless the mindset changes, that old voice in their head that tells them to react, think, and behave in familiar ways will drive them to go back to what their brain-body thinks is normal.

I know of one survivor of bariatric surgery who eats nothing but chocolate peanut butter cups and fast-food milkshakes. The mindset that convinces him that the products give him something he needs gradually overrides the surgery he experienced. And because metabolic science is science, he regained all the weight he initially lost after the surgery.

The practical changes are simple. We stop overworking the pancreas by consuming foods that are less likely to spike blood glucose levels. Thus, blood glucose levels begin to drop. Simultaneously, we begin to shift our diet toward a healthier one. (Don't assume you know what a healthier diet actually means. There is a lot of misinformation out there.) A healthier diet gives the body the fuel and nutrition it needs to heal. The body already knows *how* to heal itself.

Then we give our body time to adjust and begin to utilize the stored energy found in glycogen and body fat. We will do this by gradually extending the time between meals and later, by engaging in therapeutic, short-term, intermittent fasting. We also very gently and consistently increase our activity levels in order to address insulin resistance and speed up our metabolism.

All these steps are addressed in this book and I assure you, they are easier than you think. Especially if you take one step at a time. But there are a few things you need to understand so that you can better stick with the program and not make common mistakes.

Micronutrients vs. Macronutrients

Stroll down the vitamin supplement aisle at your local pharmacy or peruse a catalog and you might be overwhelmed by the variety of supplements available to you. The very existence of this aisle and the proliferation of supplement companies give testimony to the heart of the problems incurred by ingesting manufactured, processed food products.

Yet, the promises these supplements make are likely inflated and the quality may be questionable. While the body might benefit from supplements to deliver essential micronutrients that may be lacking in our food, a pill, gummy or capsule are not ideal ways of introducing those nutrients to the body.

It shouldn't surprise you to know that if you eat a healthy diet, you'll get most, if not all the micronutrients your body needs to thrive. As you develop your healthy lifestyle, you may discover the utility of some supplementation based on your food choices, but the needs are likely to be so few that you should not mind paying a bit more for reliable supplements of verifiable quality.

Micronutrients are not a subject we will cover in this book.

I started off this chapter talking about micronutrients so that I could contrast them with *macro*nutrients. There are only three and of the three, only two of them are necessary for a healthy life.

Carbohydrates

Carbohydrates form the basis of the standard dietary recommendations offered by governments around the world. These consist of sugar, fruit, grains such as corn, wheat, and oats, beans, and legumes, as well as starchy sugary vegetables like potatoes, carrots, and beets. Carbohydrates are cheap to produce in mass quantities and have the reputation of being able to feed the world inexpensively.

No matter how complex or simple a carbohydrate is (whole grain bread vs. white bread, for example) carbohydrates are turned into glucose by the body. The only real difference is the rate of that conversion which only slightly depends on the degree to which the grain has been processed. The more processed the quicker glucose is made. There isn't really much difference between slices of whole grain and white bread. If you were walking through a wheat field and plucked a head of wheat and just ate it, raw and encased in all that structurally complete plant fiber, it would have less effect than a slice of bread. But it would still be converted into glucose. A diet based on carbohydrates results in more blood glucose than most people can reasonably use.

The result, as we learned in the last chapter, is increased blood insulin levels. When insulin levels are chronically high—a condition known as hyperinsulinemia—the cells develop insulin resistance because they can't use all of the glucose their diet supplies. This has created a societal epidemic of metabolic diseases.

Carbohydrates, believe it or not, are completely unnecessary for human health. There may be people who need carbohydrates for some obscure medical reasons, but none, not even elite athletes, come immediately to mind. We certainly like them but the need is not there. The body can get all that it needs from the other two macronutrients. That being said, The Onesta Process is not a zero-carbohydrate program. We reduce them but not eliminate them.

Humans evolved on diets based on fat and protein. Carbohydrates were part of our evolutionary diet but they were most often sweet, limited, seasonal treats such as berries or fruit. With the advent of agriculture, humans found ways of cultivating grains so that they didn't have to search them out or stumble upon them in their food-gathering habits. Even then, the amount of grain available was limited.

Proteins

Proteins, such as meat, fish, eggs, and poultry formed the cornerstone of our evolutionary diet. We were hunter-gatherers. We hunted animals and gathered what we could as we moved from place to place. Agriculture and animal husbandry enabled us to stop wandering and live a more predictable and stable life. However, we must remember that even then, most families and groups operated at a subsistence level.

It may surprise you to know that your body can and will produce glucose from meat. About 30% of the proteins found in animal products are used as protein. The rest is converted into glucose. We can see this illustrated clearly by considering the level of blood glucose rise after consuming carbohydrates compared to proteins. The effect of proteins on blood glucose levels is significantly less than that of carbohydrates. Additionally, because it takes more to digest meat than carbohydrates, the process is slower and more controlled. These two factors help regulate the amount of insulin required to direct glucose out of the blood and into cells, giving our body a healthier time in which to process what we have eaten.

Less glucose means less insulin is required. Lowering insulin levels is the key to allowing your body to begin to heal. Your body can heal itself when you allow it to do what it wants to do, rather than what you have been forcing it to do by following a dietary regimen that is arguably unhealthy.

Fats

The final macronutrient we need to discuss is perhaps the most important and the one we have been trained to fear the most: fat. We have been told for perhaps the last 50 years that saturated fat is the root cause of heart disease. Consuming a diet high in animal fat may cause elevated levels of cholesterol but cholesterol is not the key risk indicator of cardiovascular disease.

If You Are Vegetarian or Vegan

The principles of the Onesta process rely heavily on increasing protein and healthy fat along with plenty of fresh, organic, above-ground vegetables and gradually decreasing reliance on carbohydrates, effectively undoing the damage of Key's hypothesis. The process does not advocate a high protein or even a high-fat diet, but rather seeks to restore the balance of a moderate protein and moderate fat lifestyle.

Vegetarians and vegans can benefit from therapeutic intermittent fasting, covered later, but may have difficulty achieving the reduced levels of carbohydrates and increased healthy fats that are essential for the program.

As a vegetarian or vegan, your ability to apply the principles of this program will require more work on your part because many plant-based sources of protein also come with significant levels of carbohydrates. If you are going to consume soy or gluten *products,* such as seitan and textured vegetable protein (TVP) as your main source of protein, at least consider organic sources.

It is also important to understand that plant-based proteins have approximately half the absorption rate as protein by the body than protein from animal sources. Only about 17% of plant-based protein is absorbed by the body as protein. The rest is converted into glucose.

If you can eat eggs, cheese, and/or fish, you'll have an easier time finding protein that doesn't come with a high carbohydrate cost. Other sources of vegetarian protein are often highly processed foods. It is a compromise you must be willing to make in order to maintain your vegetarian ethic. I personally do not recommend this compromise as processed foods may not be recognized by the body as real, natural, wholesome foods. On the other hand, I'd rather a vegetarian or vegan get sufficient protein to maintain their body while controlling the negative effects of carbohydrates.

Vegetarian or vegan sources of healthy fat are limited. Many of the health promises put forth about mono- and polyunsaturated oils lack definitive scientific evidence of benefit, and there are often deleterious or negative consequences of relying on these oils.

Extra virgin olive oil is a mono-unsaturated fat but despite all the Mediterranean diet cooks out there, it is not good for cooking. Like seed oils, Olive oil is easily oxidized when it is heated. As a condiment, however, and used in salad dressing, fresh extra virgin olive oil reaches perfection. If you need a liquid oil to be used in cooking, expeller extracted avocado oil is a good choice. You can always use saturated fats for cooking. Saturated fats are often solid at room temperature. The vegan source of saturated fat, the good fat, is organic, unrefined coconut oil.

Vegetable oils that have been injected with hydrogen, making them solid at room temperature are called trans fats. These fats, margarine, and vegetable shortening are toxic.

I am not some carnivore out to mock vegans and vegetarians. In fact, I was a lacto-ovo vegetarian for nearly 20 years. In 1992, I saw a nutritionist to lose weight. We followed the traditional reduced-calorie, low-fat advice still used by many today. I lost about 30 pounds. It was about then I opted for vegetarianism, as I was not eating much meat anyway and I was rather put off by industrial husbandry.

As I was advised, my diet relied heavily on grains, vegetables, and restricted fat. I only consumed the white of the eggs for protein, avoiding yolks because of the cholesterol. At the time, the supermarket shelves were filled with products labeled "fat-free." I even became quite good at baking all sorts of delicious things without fat.

After achieving my goal and basically remaining low-fat, the thirty pounds I had lost became the 100 pounds I gradually gained. After that, no matter how hard I tried, I could never achieve those results again. Based on the research, I now fully attribute both my obesity and my diabetes to that diet and the subsequent low-fat, high-carb lifestyle.

If You Are Diabetic

If you have been diagnosed with Type 2 diabetes or prediabetes, you are probably taking medications to keep your blood sugar levels in check. It is extremely important that you aggressively and consistently monitor your blood glucose levels because your medications have been designed to control those levels. As you begin to control your own blood glucose levels through diet, activity, and fasting, you run the risk of experiencing low blood sugar levels that can be quite dangerous.

Low blood sugar levels can result in unconsciousness and even death. If you are using insulin or taking medications that may lower your blood sugar levels, testing more frequently is of the utmost importance. You should keep food or juice handy to quickly counteract low blood sugar levels should that become necessary.

Your physician should be involved in any changes to your medication levels. It is likely that those medications will need to be adjusted as you progress through the program. Know that rapid changes may not be reflected in your A1c results unless you have seen consistently reduced levels for three months.

I address the concerns of those with Type 2 diabetes more extensively in my book *Life Without Diabetes*. Before progressing, I urge you to consider using that book instead of this one. The processes are virtually identical but *Life Without Diabetes* more consistently and directly addresses the concerns of a person who is reversing diabetes as well as losing weight.

Chapter Four: Toward a New Normal

The Onesta Process is not merely about reaching your target weight. It is much more than that. It is about establishing new patterns of attitude and behavior, a new lifestyle. In fact, it is about creating a new "normal" in your life.

I have heard countless people say, "I wish I could be like so-and-so. They can eat whatever they want, and never gain a pound." It is not a fair comparison, but my guess is that if we compared apples to apples, we would find significant differences in the things they want to eat and the frequency with which they eat them. This program is as much about changing what you *want* to eat as it is about changing what you eat and when.

Do not be envious of people who eat a lot of junk food and still appear fit. Outward appearances can be deceiving. Despite looking fit, many of them have fat stored behind their abdominal wall, around the organs—a condition labeled **T**hin on the **O**utside but **F**at on the **I**nside (TOFI). These unfortunate folks are often ignorant of the negative influence of metabolic disease in their lives, but they are equally susceptible to the deleterious symptomatic conditions of the disease.

Remember, above all, this one simple fact: The way we lived before we started this process, what we ate and how often we ate it, is what caused the very thing we now want to change. We have to think and behave differently for the rest of our lives to change the rest of our lives. Our relationship with food must change. That change doesn't mean we no longer enjoy what we eat, but rather that we enjoy food that doesn't slowly destroy our health.

Most people are looking for an easy way out. They want a magic pill, a superfood, a piece of equipment, a prepackaged meal, a convenient product like a milkshake, protein bar, or a dietary supplement that will resolve their problem. These products represent billion-dollar industries, and there is no end to them because none of them actually work over the long term. People just move from gimmick to gimmick, hoping that it will work and feeling guilty for failure or short-lived results.

You are beginning a process that is designed for permanent change. It addresses both the mind and the body, thus facilitating the necessary adjustments to your lifestyle. The Onesta Process is not just a plan. It is not just a program. It is a life-long process.

There are people who say they want to lose weight, but what they really mean is, if you will forgive the cliché, they want to have their cake and eat it, too. They want to eat all the things they want to eat but without the consequences. They want a better life without actually working to change the one they have. No one escapes the consequences of following the standard dietary recommendations, not even skinny people. The major causes of death in our society, including heart disease and cancer, are dietary related diseases. It's time to stop dreaming and begin to create our new normal.

We know that restricted calorie diets do not work in the long term and may well cause increasing damage to our bodies. We know that dieters lose and gain the same pounds repeatedly and eventually just give up. We know that exercise does not burn enough calories to make a real difference. Actually it is often counterproductive because results are minimal, slow in coming, and demotivating. And we leave the gym, step off the elliptical, or finish our workout with driving hunger.

It seems cruel to say, but your normal is normal. The way you are right now, your weight, your blood pressure, your cardiovascular risk, your cancer, or any other related challenges you face *are normal*. That's why you need a new normal. Your body is doing the best it can under the given circumstances. As long as you keep doing what you are doing, or going back to what you did before, what is normal for you cannot permanently change. When we change the circumstances and maintain those changes, our normal will change.

It's not fair. You have probably been doing what you and many other people think is the *right* thing to do. You have probably been following the advice you have been given as best you can. No one is perfect, and no one gets it exactly right. Instead of feeling guilty or blaming yourself for failure, reconsider the advice you have been given. Let it go and learn.

Why are there more obese and diabetic people today than there were even twenty years ago? For these two conditions to affect so many people, the cause cannot be individual responsibility. It certainly isn't the result of occasional overindulgence. It has to be something bigger.

Simply put, I believe that the epidemic levels of obesity and diabetes are the natural result of a food culture shift that began more than forty years ago, with standardized dietary recommendations based on foods that naturally spike blood glucose and create an environment of hyperinsulinemia. You might recognize it as the food pyramid. Published in 1980, we were told to cut out fat and base our diet on grains.

As a result of following that advice, your mind and body have naturally settled into its current condition. What you see in the mirror right now and the numbers that appear on your scale are normal for you, within the context of the dietary environment that we have been brainwashed to believe is healthy.

The good news is that with a bit of education, gradual adjustments, and perhaps a bit of determination, you can change that environment. And, if you maintain that change long enough, your mind and body will adjust to *a new normal*, making the results you have achieved permanent.

Your current normal is the reason you keep re-gaining the weight. Get it out of your head that the changes we will make are somehow temporary. Most of them will be permanent. There will be more wiggle room in your future, but you won't want to wiggle as much as you think you might. This is because *you* will have changed.

As we go through the process, divest yourself of the deprivation mentality. Diets by nature are restrictive. You can have *this* and you can't have *that*. It is our nature to focus on what we can't have. That pattern of thinking doesn't work in the Onesta Process. You can have anything you want. The Onesta Process helps us change what we *want*, not what we can or cannot have.

A client I was working with kept using the language of deprivation. "I know I can't eat that." Or, "I know I shouldn't eat that." At a critical point in our session, I stopped him and asked, "How old are you?"

"Sixty-seven."

"At sixty-seven, can you eat any damned thing you want?"

He stopped, thought for a minute, and said, "Yes."

Then stop telling yourself that you can't or shouldn't

eat anything. All you are doing is hypnotizing yourself into believing your life is restricted. People in prison want to get out, even if they have no idea how to behave when they do. People who tell themselves they can't eat something want to eat it more. You are sabotaging your own success. From this point forward, you will choose what you eat and what you don't eat. My job is to tell you how those decisions may affect you so that you can make better choices. If you eat something that goes against your long-term objective of losing weight, all it will do is slow you down and delay or perhaps sabotage the reaching of your goals. Is it worth eating or not?

If and when you find yourself battling between wanting to eat something and knowing that it doesn't fit, consider winning the battle with this mind hack. Tell yourself, out loud if necessary, "Even though I want to eat it, I choose to not want to eat it. I realize I do not really want to eat it, no matter how good it looks (sounds, smells) because eating it is contrary to the lifestyle I really want. It isn't worth eating, now." Notice the *now* at the end of that declaration. *Now* is temporary. There may be a time much later, after you have established your new normal, when you do choose to eat that food. If you do, however, you will discover the glamor of the food wasn't real. It won't taste as good as you thought it would and your desire to eat it again will greatly diminish.

When you make decisions about what you choose to eat, you may, for a while, make more drastic choices in order to achieve your goals more quickly. The main reason we make gradual progress during our work together is so that you become comfortable with most of those decisions, to the point of even preferring them. This process makes those choices more natural for you, and you establish your new normal. We will sustain that new condition long enough for your mind and body to recognize it as normal.

After you achieve your new normal, you may choose, once again, to occasionally eat a food or just try a food you have eliminated during the program. But the one thing that will not change is that you will always make informed decisions about what you eat.

As an illustration, when I decided to begin this program in my own life, I loved desserts. I'd never leave a wedding before they cut the cake. Since reaching my goals and maintaining them, I have sometimes tried a forkful of a dessert. That one bite is consistently too sweet for me, to the point of spitting it out into a napkin. I know a forkful of dessert isn't going to make me diabetic again, though lots of forkfuls might do so eventually. The distaste is not psychological. My taste preferences have changed. I'm no longer tempted to eat desserts, no matter how beautifully they are presented. I honestly do not *want* to eat them.

Some people believe that their normal is established by genetics. "Everyone in my family is fat. What chance do I have?" We recognize that genes allow for certain potential conditions. It was once hoped that genetic modification might actually cure diseases. As it turns out, we do not have to actually modify our genes; we can turn them on and off. The science of epigenetics, which demonstrates that the function of genes can be influenced by their environment, indicates that lasting change is possible. Your new normal will be that new environment. You will change.

I label the Onesta Process as a hypnosis-facilitated lifestyle change to lose weight and control Type 2 diabetes. Anyone can make the dietary changes necessary to lose weight or to gain control over and even reverse their Type 2 diabetes. The practical steps are enough. However, in order to maintain those changes, the mind and the body need to be in harmony. To lose weight permanently, you need more than a temporary change in diet or behavior. In order for results to stick, *your mindset* also needs to change.

Many people think that changing is a difficult process, but it isn't really. Every time we learn, we change in some way. Every time we grow, we change in some way. Every time we elect to change, it goes with having learned something and having grown in some way. In this program, you will be asked to learn and to apply what you have learned. You will grow and you will change.

The biggest obstacle to change is the unconscious mind, which guides all of our automatic thoughts, behaviors, and responses. The unconscious mind is powerful. It operates on the premise that what has been working so far is useful, and changing what is useful should be resisted. Intellectually, we know that in at least one case—our relationship with food—change is necessary.

These days, smoking is generally understood as a risky behavior that can lead to cancer and an extremely uncomfortable end of life. We would be hard-pressed to find a smoker who does not intellectually know this, but the unconscious mind believes that smoking provides some benefit that has worked for years and years. An obese person may intellectually know that a donut is not really going to help them—indeed, it may harm them—but that voice in the back of their mind that says, "I need a donut," wins.

The wonderful thing about our process is that you don't have to eat your last donut. You can always choose to eat a donut and you'll have that choice available to you for the rest of your life. You probably won't exercise that choice often and it is very likely that if and when you do choose to eat a donut, it won't be the same. If you are like most of us, it will be too sweet for you. You won't like it, and the temptation will disappear. A small portion of that donut might be more than enough to satisfy your curiosity.

Think of this. Have you ever gone to a birthday party, graduation, or wedding and looked forward to the cake? Are you one of those people who ask for a small piece while wishing you could eat the entire thing? What would it feel like to celebrate that person or event in a truly heartfelt way, whether there was cake or not? Imagine how much closer you would feel to that person or the people celebrating the event when your heart was in the celebration and not the cake. In fact, you may choose not to eat the cake but rather enjoy participating in the celebration.

Hypnosis works on the unconscious mind and helps change manifest in such a way that it becomes natural, despite the prior experience. Hypnosis helps the unconscious mind integrate new information, experiences, and perceptions so that the unconscious mind changes.

Achieving results is good, but unless the unconscious mind changes as well, you'll be the same and you will gravitate back to the way things were. As long as you still think you "need" a donut, you have more work to do.

Granted, the practical information in this book will do the job. But will you follow it? Hypnosis certainly helps there. Will you stick to it? The hypnosis and the accountability of a coach guiding you through the process help. All those group weight loss programs employ that strategy. Even some of the apps, which might compare your results to others in the program or encourage your participation in chat groups, attempt the same thing.

Here's the critical question: Will you still like your life during and after completing the program? What if I could promise you that you will not only like it, you will enjoy it more than you do now, and even more than you would if you achieved your goal alone?

If you choose to do it alone, I urge you not to downplay the psychological strategies or mind hacks described in this book and strongly urge you to employ self-hypnosis if you know how.

All change, even positive change, creates stress. Some of us can maintain motivation and emotional strength throughout the stress of change and do it without help. Most of us, however, need support, strategies, and tools for adapting to the changes we want to make.

Hypnosis is not magic, but it sometimes feels that way. Hypnosis gives the unconscious mind free access to new information that allows it to make changes in the patterns it has established. Hypnosis reduces anxiety, helps fight cravings, increases motivation and commitment, combats and reframes emotional eating, and even boosts the immune system—all while making you feel great.

Your unconscious mind can embrace short-term changes as a matter of survival, a way of coping with a temporary condition. We sometimes call this phenomenon willpower. It is as if the conscious mind is bullying the unconscious into temporary compliance. It's temporary, and compliance is not effective change. Instruction and coaching combined with hypnotherapy provide a three-pronged approach for real, long-lasting change that will be evidenced in your thoughts, emotions, and your body. In this program, we are teaching your body and your mind, both conscious and unconscious, to *be* different, to establish a *new normal*. In effect, we are resetting the defaults.

The most common technique, one that often works against our conscious objectives, is called self-hypnosis. In the past, every time you sabotaged your success either in dieting or exercise, you did it in a self-hypnotic trance. Can you recall talking yourself into eating something you thought you shouldn't or talking yourself out of the exercise you planned? Most people don't realize how often they use self-hypnosis. When you are working with a clinical hypnotist, the information delivered to the unconscious mind is the job of the hypnotist. In self-hypnosis, the unconscious mind and the conscious mind are in effect duking it out. You can more easily control your conscious mind than your unconscious mind. Taking the initiative and putting in the effort to do that is often critical to the success of the change work.

When some people hear the term self-hypnosis, they think of listening to recordings or a kind of focused meditation exercise. You can, of course, utilize recorded hypnosis sessions. The best are customized and recorded specifically for you. Usually, these are offered as a service by the hypnotist and are simply a recording of a completed session. I allow my clients to record our sessions to their phones when we are working in person and allow them to record the session to their computers if we are working online.

I encourage them to only listen to those recordings as if we were repeating the session and not listen to them casually. We don't want to take a successful session that reaches the unconscious mind and bring it to the completely conscious level. The conscious mind can act like a filter and perhaps undo some of what the hypnosis session accomplished.

I also caution them to not share the recording with others for two reasons. First, the session was customized and specific to the particular needs or concerns of the client. The second, I admit, is selfish. It's not about money. I don't charge for the recordings, but the recordings lack the disclaimer to not do something silly like listening to the recording while driving.

If you are experienced at working with a hypnotist, you'll do better at achieving the kind of self-hypnosis that is a form of meditation. The more often you are hypnotized, the better you are at going into a hypnotic trance. You may find it easier to control your mind, relax into the session, and allow your unconscious mind to absorb notions or ideas that can help facilitate the change. Without experience, however, achieving that level of focus and concentration can prove difficult.

With my clients, I provide them with a recording of my standard induction. Both my voice and the words are familiar to them. If they want to change the content of the focus of their self-hypnosis exercise, they can stipulate the purpose and intent of the session before beginning the recording. Intentions should always be expressed in a positive way. "I am going to practice self-hypnosis for the purpose of feeling calm and peaceful." Rather than negatively, "I am going to practice self-hypnosis for the purpose of not being so anxious and worried." A positive intention is focused on a defined goal rather than a negative one focused on getting away from some condition or problem.

After a number of sessions, I will actually teach my clients how to enter trance on their own, without a recording. By that time, they are both focused on what they want and are familiar enough with hypnosis to know that they are actually hypnotized. If time is limited, I tell them to set an alarm in their mind, "I'm going to practice self-hypnosis for 15 minutes for the purpose of feeling refreshed and energized." The internal clock can be quite useful for alarms. Failing that, I instruct them to simply set a practical alarm in case they fall asleep.

All of the above buy into the standard understanding of self-hypnosis, but there is a very powerful form of self-hypnosis that is almost always in play. Your unconscious mind is always trying to prompt you into action—*or inaction*—by injecting thoughts, reactions, or automatic behaviors that reinforce your status quo, your current normal. It does this automatically and frankly does not consider your conscious desire to change.

The default setting of your unconscious mind is your current normal, whatever it is. If you have ever asked yourself why you repeatedly do something or why you always end up feeling a certain way, this is due to the default settings of your unconscious mind.

For about five years, I was involved in consumer education and worked on a program that helped restore banking privileges to folks who had bounced so many checks that the banks closed their accounts and reported them to a system that would prohibit other banks from offering them a checking account. People in this situation often blame the banks for their condition. "The bank bounced my checks." But let's face it, if a problem keeps repeating itself for someone, the real cause is much closer to home. The source of that problem is likely an unconscious emotion, thought, reaction, or behavior. How often have you said to yourself, "I know I shouldn't _____, but..."

In this process, you are changing your normal—psychologically, physiologically, and emotionally—to one that does not accommodate obesity. In effect, you are resetting your defaults. In doing so, you are choosing new ones.

For a while, it will be like running a neck-to-neck race. The practical steps you wish to employ will compete with those automatic thoughts, reactions, and emotions. Every time you feel tempted to cheat on the process, the thought to do so has come from your unconscious mind. The thought is a hypnotic suggestion trying to convince you to maintain homeostasis, or the status quo. When you actually cheat, you are sabotaging yourself in a self-hypnotic state.

The trick to dealing with self-sabotage is to recognize the thought or temptation *and* the situation or circumstance that triggered it. We'll talk a bit more about the triggers when we talk about hunger, cravings, and emotional eating. Suffice it to say now that when you recognize the thought, the best form of self-hypnosis aimed at changing your unconscious mind is to correct the thought. In effect, you will rewrite or reword the thought to reflect the opposite intention.

The thought *I am starving* is nothing short of a lie. If you are interested in this process, you certainly are not starving. Chances are there is enough fat on your body that you are nowhere near starving in the strictest sense of the word. You *feel* hungry, perhaps intensely so, but it is a feeling, not a condition. Catch the thought and stop it. Instead of focusing on a hunger pang, stop, and consider the situation, circumstance, or environment in which the pang emerged. Rewrite the thought to something like, *I'm perfectly fine and will easily wait for dinner.*

I admit that sometimes pulling off this kind of self-hypnosis is a challenge, but we must realize that our current situation is due to the lifestyle we have been living. We have to admit that, at least in some respects, we've gotten it wrong and we have to correct ourselves. It is best to accomplish that from the inside out.

In the next chapter, I present the initial stage of the Onesta Process. After that, every other chapter will focus on either topics relevant to the process or the following stages of it. After the first stage, which should last a week, you can remain at any stage for up to several weeks before going on to the next. When you feel comfortable with that change, move on to the next. You can read the topical chapters as you work through the program or if it so happens, when they apply to you.

Chapter Five: Stage One

———— ❧ ————

Set Your Baseline

In this first stage, we will primarily focus on getting ready to start the program. Learning to swim provides a good analogy. Few swimming instructors would throw an adult learner into the middle of the deep end of the pool on the first day. Since I do not know what you know or what you think, it is best for us to proceed more methodically. In this stage, we will cover some basic information, learn how to track our progress and make a single major change in the way we eat. That is it.

First things first. Take a full-body "before" picture. When you see your "after" picture, you'll be glad you did. If you don't like having your picture taken, then you'll take a bad picture. But if you want to feel good about the picture, smile, step forward, make yourself larger than life, and pose. Stretch your arms out in a posture that says, "Hey! I'm here and glad to be here." Think of that phrase when you take the picture, and you'll take a better picture. The pose looks silly in real life, but in the photo, it won't. I promise.

At a time convenient for you, preferably just after you wake up, step on the scale and see how much you weigh. In a journal or diary or even the calendar on your phone, note your weight. This is your starting point. Be honest.

Do not weigh yourself every day. Your body weight can fluctuate by any number of pounds from day to day. I recommend you weigh yourself no more frequently than every two weeks. I ask my clients to weigh themselves only on the days of our appointments.

Also, get a tape measure, like those made of cloth that are used for sewing, and measure your waist at the navel. Don't use the waist size of your pants. It may not be an accurate measure. Different manufacturers cut their clothing differently. And many large people wear their trousers a bit tight in the waist and have a bit of a muffin top, often hidden by an untucked shirt. Let's measure our waist size for real, shall we? If there are other measurements you are interested in, note them. Men often like to use their neck size because that is how they buy dress shirts.

The reason for the different measurements is twofold.

First, waist size is considered an indicator of metabolic syndrome. Second, different people experience results in different ways. Your body shape may change before the scale reflects a weight change, or vice versa. Measure yourself no more often than every two weeks and don't be discouraged if your body resists changing at first.

A few of my weight loss clients have elected to test their blood glucose levels voluntarily because they are a good indicator of insulin levels. Doing so is not necessary but go ahead if you are one of those folks who like to track data. Get a meter and have at it. You can buy them over the counter. Often, the fastest results are seen in blood glucose levels. We are interested in the first reading of the day, just before your first bite of food or sip of anything other than water. Write those numbers down and average them out just before beginning stage two.

Your First Steps

Set aggressive goals. If you are like most dieters, you've been trained to set modest goals because achieving them seems motivating. On the other hand, if you achieve a modest goal, how likely are you to be able to maintain motivation if you really want to go farther? I encourage my client to set an aggressive goal, explaining that it is easier to stop if you feel satisfied along the way, but mustering up the motivation to go beyond a modest goal is both difficult and discouraging. Go for the aggressive goal. Think about your ideal weight and the kind of lifestyle you want to live. Look up the ideal weight for your height online and subtract another five pounds. Take a moment to close your eyes and imagine what it will be like to be you when you achieve your goal. What will your life look like? What will you look like? What will you do for fun?

I once attended a "vision quest" seminar in which we were encouraged to establish goals and then create a collage out of magazine pictures that represented those goals. I don't think much of my collage manifested in my life at the time, mostly because my goals evolved. I learned a lot about myself through the process. The collage sat above my desk for a long time. The important thing is that it motivated me to continue growing and becoming my more authentic self. I strongly recommend doing something like this because the journey ahead may be a long one.

We will only make small changes during stage one. The first is to *only eat from a bowl or plate*, and the second is to *take a picture of everything you eat*. If you are having a snack, plate it and take a picture of it. No more snacking from a bag or box. If you want more than you have plated, put more on the plate and take another picture. Keep the pictures in a file or gallery labeled Stage One. My clients send their pictures to me the day before our next session. We do this task only for the first three or four sessions. After that, there's no need, but the pictures serve a very real purpose.

When clients hear the instruction to take pictures of everything they eat, they assume that we are looking for habits of overeating. Often they have been dieting on and off—sometimes continuously—for many years, and the message of "eat less, exercise more" has been drummed into their minds. Because they are still overweight, they assume they are overeating and not exercising enough.

My experience is that the opposite is true. I find that people who have been habituated to dieting do not eat enough. They might unconsciously snack, and the plating of snacks points out the snacking, but when we look at those pictures of meals, I am more often than not looking for ways of *increasing* what they have on their plate. If you are not eating enough, your body is in semi-starvation mode.

I also use these pictures to identify the carbohydrates on the plate. What we have been told is healthy eating—limited quantities of lean meat and a reliance on "complex" carbohydrates—is often what my obese clients are faithfully eating. The reduction in fat leaves people feeling hungry. Fat stimulates leptin, the hormone that indicates satiety. Fat also provides a mechanism for fat-soluble nutrients to be easily absorbed. As a consequence, a low-fat diet reduces satiety and inhibits proper nutrition, causing hunger.

Unless you are picking raw stalks of grain and eating them whole, there really is no such thing as a carbohydrate sufficiently complex enough to make a significant difference. Certainly, eating complex carbohydrates is better than eating simple carbohydrates and sugars, but the delay in digesting even the most complex carbohydrates on the general market is insignificant because of the processing.

You'll digest milled grain more quickly than if you ate the whole seeds. Raw sugar is still sugar.

You should remove distractions while you eat. Many people eat unconsciously. I don't mean they aren't aware that they're eating. Rather, they occupy their minds with something other than eating while they eat. They might eat at their computer. Some will scroll through their phones and check their email or social media feeds. Remove all distractions from your meal.

Sit down to eat. Don't eat standing up or on the run. It may seem silly, but before you begin eating, use that internal monologue voice to tell your body, "I'm going to eat now." Many people say grace before eating. It's a wonderful way of signaling to your body that it's time to eat. In Japan, they signal the beginning of a meal by saying *itadakimasu*; in France, bon appétit. It doesn't have to be a religious thing. Just focus your attention on eating when you sit down to eat, and do nothing else while eating. If you notice your mind wandering while eating, bring it back to your plate and focus your attention on the flavor and texture of your food.

The last but very important thing we are doing during stage one is establishing your average *natural fast*. Unless you eat while you are sleeping, you are fasting from some point in the evening until some point the next day. You break that fast with the first sip or bite that contains either carbohydrates or protein. We'll discount fat because of its low impact on blood glucose and insulin. Coffee with a splash of heavy cream—not milk, not soy or oat milk—doesn't break the fast.

Track the times when you take your last bite one day and your first bite the next. Calculate the hours. Write the hours down every day for a week, and at the end of the week, add them up and divide them by the number of days you tracked. This is your average natural fast. I'll tell you what to do with that number in stage two.

At this point, you are still looking to see if this program will work. If keeping these records seems onerous, you would benefit from working with a hypnotist trained in the science and coaching of this program. Accountability makes compliance easier. Most of us work in person, locally or long-distance over the internet. To find a hypnotist coach, visit **www.onestaprocess.com**.

Whether you are working alone or with a certified hypnotist coach, you'll need to understand the following information.

Macronutrients Revisited

Very few foods actually fit snugly into a single macronutrient category. Most deliver more than one macronutrient in varying percentages. In our process, we are mostly interested in the main or dominant macronutrient in a food or menu item. Bread, for example, is primarily a carbohydrate, but contains some protein in the form of gluten. Bread also often contains some fat. Olives are considered fat but contain some carbohydrates. While we are primarily concerned with the dominant macronutrient of a particular food, we must keep in mind that other macronutrients come in the package, especially in terms of carbohydrates.

Recall that each macronutrient is processed by the body differently and thus has a different effect on blood glucose and the consequential insulin secretion. This fact is also one of the essential reasons that understanding body weight as a mere factor of calories is doomed to failure. Fat carries the highest number of calories per gram. Of the three macronutrient categories, it contains nearly twice the calories per gram as protein or carbohydrates. However, fat has the least effect on blood glucose and insulin levels. Since insulin is a critical part of the process of storing glucose as fat (thus increasing body fat), dietary fat has little to no effect on weight gain.

One does not have to think very hard about how dietary macronutrients can affect blood glucose levels in an insulin-resistant or diabetic person. People who are not diabetic (yet?) have a pancreas that has been up to the task of managing blood glucose thus far. If they are overweight, we know that excess glucose is being directed to the liver and is being converted into fat. However, in a person with elevated levels of blood glucose, the pancreas is showing signs of not being as effective. This reduction in effectiveness is likely due to the constant deluge of carbohydrates and sugars into the bloodstream. A less likely cause may be that damage has been done to the pancreas. In either case, consuming foods that do not increase the need for elevated insulin levels will be helpful.

Carbohydrates have nearly twice the glucose response of protein, despite having the same number of calories per gram. Protein has a moderate effect on blood glucose. Fat has a negligible impact on blood glucose.

When these factors are taken into consideration, obesity can easily be seen as a result of consuming too many carbohydrates, no matter how healthy the package claims them to be.

In your research, you may discover something called resistant starch. These are carbohydrates whose impact on blood glucose is slightly more controlled. There is a suspicion that products high in carbohydrates can be made "resistant" by treating them differently, often by freezing them. I've seen such conflicting information on this later hypothesis that I am reluctant to place any stock in it.

In this program, those testing their blood glucose levels will have the opportunity to see which foods have the highest impact on their own blood sugar levels. People who do not want to reduce carbs are always looking for ways of cheating the system. As my mother would have said, "They want to have their cake and eat it, too."

You'll get farther in the program if you understand that you aren't being asked to *eliminate* carbohydrates from your diet. Instead, you are being challenged to be savvy about which carbohydrates you choose and how much of them you consume. We intend to reduce our carbohydrate consumption because of the effect they have on our bodies. The amount of the reduction depends on you and the condition of your body. Some will make very dramatic reductions, while others will only reduce those significant enough to achieve their objectives. You will always be in charge of which carbohydrates you choose to eat and how much of them you consume.

Over the next week:

- Eat normally. Eat what you normally eat when you normally eat it, but...

- Plate everything you eat, even snacks.

- Take a picture of every plate. You might want to make notes if you don't eat everything on the plate. When viewing photos with clients, they will often comment on what they did and did not eat on the plate, especially when the meal was in a restaurant. While taking pictures of your food may seem silly or even punitive, it is the best way to see how your eating plan is changing. You need to do that.

- Eat intentionally, without distractions. Don't do anything else while you eat.

- Track your natural fast from the last caloric bite or sip in the evening to the first bite or sip the next day. Calculate your average natural fast.

- And, if you are testing your blood glucose, take a blood glucose reading just prior to your first bite or sip. Note the readings and calculate your average blood glucose at the end of the week.

One week at this stage should be sufficient to set your baseline. Make sure you record all the information. At the end of the week, calculate your averages. Do not weigh yourself again until the first day of stage two.

Chapter Six: Hunger, Cravings, and Emotional Eating

Handling Hunger

The sensation of hunger is tied to a hormone called *ghrelin*. When ghrelin is produced, we feel hungry. A sense of satiety, or being satisfied, is associated with another hormone called *leptin*. These hormones may be stimulated by physical, mental, or emotional conditions. A memory that makes you feel angry is stimulating hormones. A stressful situation is stimulating hormones. Stubbing your toe stimulates hormones. Once we make a mind-body association between eating or hunger and some other condition, every time we experience the condition, we will eat without thinking. If eating is delayed, we are likely to feel hungry until we do. That is, unless we rewire those associations.

It is helpful to understand the conditions that cause our hunger pangs. We all differ a little in this. Believe it or not, unless you are a high-performance athlete, the most common triggers for hunger have nothing to do with the need for energy or nutrients. For example, the rumbling in your stomach that you associate with hunger is nothing more than what you have already eaten being moved through your digestive tract.

Hunger does not grow the longer you don't eat. In fact, it dissipates. People who fast beyond a certain amount of time universally claim that they do not feel hungry. It is not a mind game. It takes time to reach the point of true hunger, and we are unlikely to fast that long in the process outlined in this book. As we proceed, the better you will understand the sources of hunger, and the more manageable hunger will become.

Hunger may be triggered by a lack of energy in the case of elite athletes and a lack of nutrition in the case of obese people whose low-fat diets primarily consist of carbohydrates. However, for most of us, most of the time, the feeling of hunger is an interpretation of an experience, a thought, or an emotion. In fact, we most often feel hunger as a habit. That is, we get hungry when we think it is time to eat. Some of us constantly feel hungry because we have grown accustomed to grazing or snacking all day long.

What we call "hunger" is really just an urge to eat, and that urge comes from many possible triggers. Hunger is often an automatic response and, though our bodies may not be hungry, we *feel* hungry. That feeling may range from simply a peckish desire to nibble to a frantic ravenous drive.

We feel hungry if the clock is approaching our normal mealtimes. Eating at certain times of the day is a matter of habit, and we have trained our bodies to expect to eat at those times. If we create a habit of going to the vending machine at work during the mid-afternoon, we'll feel hungry as that time approaches. Habitual hunger happens even if our body doesn't need energy or nutrition.

The mind and the body like patterns because it is through patterns that normalcy is established. We are going to upset that pattern for a while and teach our body not to depend on time or any other trigger to decide when eating is appropriate, at least not before we reach our goals.

Over the last 30 or 40 years, our society has shifted from eating three square meals a day to eating those meals and casually snacking in between. Many of us graze throughout the day. The result is almost a constant feeling of hunger. As a society, we are almost always ready to eat, and when we are not eating, we feel a bit hungry. I have had clients tell me that they had no idea what it meant to feel full or satisfied.

There was a time when children were routinely denied a snack after school because it might *ruin their dinner*. Now, more commonly, kids snack to tide themselves over until dinner. How absurd! No matter how active kids are, they can occupy themselves for two or three hours until dinner time. And since most of those snacks are carbohydrates, processed foods, and sugary snacks, they'd be far better off without them.

In our new lifestyle, we will teach our bodies to get ready to eat when we sit down to eat. In fact, we have already started. Remember that from this point forward, when you eat, you should do it *intentionally*, without distractions like the television, your phone, or a book. Set a place at the table, eat off of plates, and focus on your food.

We may feel hungry when our blood sugar drops, especially if it does so precipitously. There used to be a commercial that suggested a candy bar was the perfect mid-afternoon snack to tide one over until dinner. Anyone who has ever tried that likely found themselves back at the vending machine as little as ten minutes after eating the candy. The reason is that the candy bar, mostly sugar, created a rapid increase in blood glucose levels that was naturally followed by an increase in insulin. Recall that the job of insulin is to get glucose out of the blood and direct it into cells that need it. A strong spike in blood glucose demands a heavy dose of insulin. Down come the blood glucose levels, and the drop may well trigger feelings of hunger. I call this carbohydrate hunger. It can also happen one to two hours after a meal.

That feeling of carbohydrate hunger doesn't necessarily indicate that blood glucose levels are low. Indeed, people with high blood glucose levels still experience it. It just indicates that the blood glucose levels have dropped from the spike. Stop spiking your blood glucose, and feelings of hunger will be less common and less dramatic.

The feeling of hunger can be triggered by the smell of certain foods or the sight of other appetizing items. Even the thoughts and memories we have can trigger feelings of hunger or cravings. We may feel hungry in response to certain emotions.

It becomes important for us to identify the triggers of hunger that dominate our experience. One client admitted to being a stress eater: "When I was working remotely through Covid, I noticed that every time I felt pressure in my work, I'd get up from the computer and, without thinking, open the refrigerator. I didn't have a refrigerator at my office so I hadn't noticed this trend until Covid. I wasn't really hungry but the stress was telling me to eat something."

Real hunger is not merely having an empty stomach. In fact, throughout history, human stomachs have often, even routinely been empty. From early humans who ate only when they found or successfully hunted food, to well within the last 100 years, people simply lived with an empty stomach until food was available. I keep thinking about those old movies where farm hands stopped working when the sound of a triangle bell told them that supper was ready. They waited *and worked* until then!

As a result of industrial agriculture, processed, prepackaged foods, and the emergence of fast and convenient foods, American society has been trained to snack and do it frequently. We eat all the time. The more we eat, the more money they make. And because of the way they manufacture their food products, the more we eat, the hungrier we get.

One of the arguments in favor of the industrialization of food is that we need the food to feed a rising population. Truth be told, upwards of 40% of the food produced in the United States is wasted. Perhaps if we consumed healthier food in healthier amounts, we wouldn't have such waste. At that rate, we could easily decrease farm intensity and sponsor more organic and humanely produced food.

Instead of sitting down to a home-cooked, whole-food dinner, we are carting Jenny off to soccer and Billy to martial arts, handing them bags of chips, cookies, yogurt, and pudding snacks to tide them over until, on the way home, we hand them a bag of something we picked up at a drive-through. That is no way to raise a healthy child with a healthy relationship with food.

Sadly, much of what we consume in the form of processed foods is so nutritionally sparse (or the enriched nutrients are not well absorbed by the body) that people in modern society are actually overfed and undernourished.

We have to learn to recognize the difference between real hunger and merely feeling hungry. The feelings of hunger pass quickly. They come and go like waves and are nothing more than a response to some stimulus that tells us it is time to eat. Feeling hungry is most often just a feeling and not a biological necessity. Let's be honest, an overweight person is not lacking sufficient fuel. In fact, they have an excess.

When you feel hungry, take a moment to observe the

feeling. Where is it in your body? We associate hunger with an empty stomach, but you might be surprised about where the feeling of hunger resides in your body. It may be in your stomach, but often it is sensed elsewhere. Some people experience it in their mouths, salivating like one of Pavlov's dogs. Sometimes it is a general sense of urgency or anxiety, often located in the chest. Sometimes it is more thirst than hunger and we are confusing the two. Sometimes, hunger can be located in your hands, expressing a need for distraction, entertainment, or occupation because it's motivated by boredom. It may be centered around the temples or feel like pressure in the forehead, as if a headache were coming on. Sometimes it is low in the gut, at the base of the spine, and may be an expression of sublimated emotions or desires.

Once you find it, just observe it for a while. Do not judge it as good or bad. Do not try to get away from it by putting something in your mouth. Do not let it make you frantic. Just observe it. What does it do? Does it change in intensity? How about in its urgency? Honestly, it may disappear entirely while you are watching it.

If you can identify the real need, address it. If you are bored, find something to do. If you are in need of comfort, comfort yourself or ask someone for a hug. If you are lonely, invite someone for a cup of coffee or tea, or simply go out and be around other people. If you are stressed, find a relaxing activity or a breathing routine to respond directly to the need, rather than following the distraction of an urge.

Crushing Cravings and Emotional Eating

We have already covered how some emotions might trigger sensations of hunger. Cravings are a little different in that they are often tied to a specific food or a specific behavior. A person might crave sweets, and it is reasonable to assume that it is not the body expressing a sugar deficiency. A person might eat compulsively, even unconsciously, finishing a family-size bag of chips in order to distract themselves from having to face feelings or situations. Another person may have the best of intentions to eat a healthy meal but refuse to plan and consequently find themselves craving fast food and making the excuse to stop at a drive-through.

While it's true that most processed, manufactured, and packaged foods come laced with sugar or a sugar derivative and other flavor enhancers, rendering them addictive, the actual cravings are often related to the convenience, the sense of having a treat, or the desire to escape life, even if only briefly enough to order and pick up a drive-through meal.

I recommend avoiding processed and manufactured food whenever possible. This means avoiding fast food and chain restaurants, buying the freshest, most organic meat and produce that one can afford, planning meals, and cooking from scratch.

It is built into human nature to be attracted to sweet things. Throughout human evolution, sweet things were rare and seasonal. When our hunter-gatherer ancestors found them, they gorged themselves, storing up a bit of extra fat for the long and lean winter ahead when fresh food was scarce and they might go for weeks without a successful hunt. If strawberries came only once a year, we'd enjoy them for a week or so and then go another year without them.

Today's fresh produce has been bred for durability in shipping and increased shelf life. It is distinctly different from the fresh fruit and vegetables that were only seasonally available for a short period of time. The reason that organic produce is so expensive relies both on the shipping, which has to be expedited due to the reduced shelf life, as well as the additional expense incurred by avoiding chemical fertilizers, pesticides, and herbicides.

In a sense, cravings for something sweet are inherently human. Given our exposure to over-sweetened foods, we have become insensitive to the sublime sweetness of an organic apple or the subtle taste profiles between two different vine-ripened heirloom tomatoes. We have in effect deadened our taste buds to anything that isn't flavor enhanced. When your taste buds become more accustomed to real food, that artificial stuff becomes repellent.

Let's get down to brass tacks about cravings. All cravings are distractions. In the instance of chemical addiction, the reduction in the amount of the chemical in the body may trigger a craving, and prolonged avoidance may encounter withdrawal. Most cravings that interest us in terms of obesity and diabetes are not really chemical addictions apart from the neurotransmitters, dopamine, serotonin, or oxytocin triggered by the *associations* with certain foods.

Apart from sugar, most foods aren't really psychoactive.

There is no real need to hack our way through a jungle of hard science here. I'm oversimplifying, but simple is enough for most folks. If you are interested in metabolic science, I suggest exploring the list of recommended reading at the end of the book. Those authors are either scientists themselves or investigative journalists of the highest repute. They extensively cite reliable scientific studies and point out the discrepancies that present themselves through the narrow focus of the scientific method. If you are a scientist and aren't afraid of diving into those studies, look up the studies those authors cite.

For our purposes, it is enough to say that dopamine is the neurotransmitter associated with pleasure. Serotonin is associated with comfort, safety, and tranquility. Oxytocin is associated with love, affection, and human connection.

When we crave a particular food, it is almost always associated with the need or desire for the feelings that are associated with these neurotransmitters because we like the way we feel when they are stimulated. Cravings are the product of the desire for those brain chemicals. Your brain-body knows about the association and creates a craving that it believes will stimulate the chemistry needed to feel better. Cravings are the very definition of emotional eating.

Imagine, for a moment, a crying baby sitting in a highchair. Mom or dad knows the baby wants attention, wants to be picked up and held, or perhaps just offloaded into a diaper. But there is too much going on at the moment. The soup is boiling, the veggies need chopping, the phone is ringing. The loving but overwhelmed parent hands the baby a cookie. Distracted by the sweet treat, the baby stops crying while the phone is answered, and the veggies are chopped.

If this pattern is repeated often enough, the baby will learn that when they are uncomfortable, no matter what the reason, the solution is eating something sweet. We're not talking about bad parenting here. It would be unfair for the baby to grow up and blame mom or dad for their emotional eating habit or their cravings for sweets. But the association can be forged at the youngest of ages.

Emotional eating and cravings usually come down to one of three functions: reward, compensation, or distraction. If we've worked exceptionally hard or have successfully navigated a tough time, we want a pat on the back. That might come in the form of a cupcake. If life has presented one disappointment after another, we may feel that we are owed a compensatory treat. Most often, however, we are simply feeling uncomfortable and want to distract ourselves from the discomfort for a little while.

If you know anyone who claims to have an "addictive personality," they most often use the object of their addiction(s) to interrupt some other feeling. It doesn't matter what the object of the addiction is, be it alcohol, drugs, sex, pornography, gambling, or sugar. The chemistry associated with giving into the addiction is more pleasant than facing and confronting the discomfort.

The essential task for the person establishing a new metabolic normal is to identify the reason they are seeking reward, compensation, or distraction. They can learn how to identify, observe, and even confront the feelings. It is true that true addictions have a chemical element of their own, but the intermingling of chemical and emotional addictions cannot be ignored. Sometimes the emotional stimulus is as simple as boredom or as complicated as the need for security or approval. Whatever the reason, the emotions are there.

I remember an occasion I've shared in a number of places, including my book *Deleting Diabetes*. While I was engaged in taking care of my elderly mother, I often stopped at the grocery store on the way to her home to get something she needed or wanted. It was an emotionally fatiguing time, and on one occasion, I treated myself to a chocolate bar, telling myself that I would only indulge in one section of the bar and save the rest for later. I remember opening the bar, placing the section into my mouth, and driving the rest of the way to my mother's house. Upon arrival, the entire candy bar was gone. I had only the vaguest memories of convincing myself that one more section wouldn't hurt.

I know why I bought the candy bar and I know why I ate it, but eating it did nothing to resolve the fatigue or the complicated emotions that confronted my life at the time.

Take cravings for what they are—unconscious distractions—and try to identify the situation you wish to forget or feel differently about. Acknowledge that the object of your craving, be it ice-cream, a pizza, or a bowl of mac and cheese, will not change the root cause of the craving.

Observe the craving. Locate it in your body. I've heard a number of fellow hypnotists assert that if you can't identify where the feeling is, how do you know you are actually feeling it? Often the inability to find the feeling in your body is related to your avoidance of it, not its lack of location. It might be in more than one place, but it has a place. Hunt it down.

Once you locate it, observe it. This is not a terribly pleasant thing to do at first, but soon enough you will begin to separate yourself from that feeling. It is like observing an obstinate, attention-seeking child throwing a tantrum. Just watch it and wait for it to lose steam. Don't try to get away from it. Observe it and wait.

If you have identified the trigger of the craving, address it in another way. If you are bored, you need something to do. If you are sad, you need to laugh. If you are lonely, you need to be around other people. And if you are feeling overwhelmed, you need to clear your head. Instead of that candy bar on the drive to my mother's house, what I really needed was to take a few moments and dedicate them to me. I might have walked around the parking lot, done a breathing exercise, or just taken time to think back and remember a time when my mother was more vibrant, more the mommy I remember as a child. None of that would have changed the actual situation, but it would have (or at least could have) changed my reaction to it. All the chocolate bar did was spike my blood sugar and make me feel guilty.

One self-hypnotic technique you can use to break the trance associated with hunger or craving is to simply get busy. Do something you enjoy or something that is purposeful but different from what you were doing when the craving cropped up. Focus your attention on accomplishing a task, especially one that you have been procrastinating about. Get stuck into that closet you want to clean out. Take your car to the car wash. Or better yet, do it by hand the old-school way.

Some folks lack the immediate ability to do what they know they need to do to confront uncomfortable feelings. If you find yourself ruminating, with your mind seeming to have a life and will of its own, you can break the trance through a simple exercise called bilateral stimulation. It may sound silly, but anything going on in your brain uses both electrical signals and chemistry. When we consciously move away from rumination and distract ourselves with something else, we effectively begin rewiring the brain, teaching it to do something other than follow an old pattern.

If you can't break the trance by getting busy, you can use a technique I often teach my clients. Pick up a small object that fits comfortably into your hands but is substantial enough to comfortably maneuver. When I teach my clients this technique, I give them a small ball, like a stress ball, but heavier. I instruct them to concentrate on the ball, not the craving, the hunger, or even the emotion they are feeling at the time.

Then, in a wide, sweeping, almost pendulum-like motion, begin handing the ball back and forth from one hand to the other. Extend the arms as you do this, all the while concentrating on the ball. When you do this, the electricity involved in the brain circuit that focuses on the craving is diverted by the tactile stimulation of the ball in their hands and the motion of their hands and arms. Passing the ball back and forth for several minutes relaxes and distracts the brain. Now they can focus their attention on other things.

You will certainly be craving carbohydrates during stages two and three because of the unusual drop in carbohydrate-based blood glucose levels. Your liver may well have begun using more glycogen to keep your levels normal while your brain started craving the carbohydrates that normally do the job. If your blood glucose numbers haven't changed, don't be discouraged. Your body is now beginning to do what it was designed to do.

A Note on Eating Disorders

Most clinical hypnotists are not qualified to diagnose or treat actual eating disorders. We can often help with the mitigation of urges, but in most cases, we are not licensed mental health professionals. I have worked with a number of mental health practitioners who thought their clients would benefit from the complementary practice of hypnosis. If you have a diagnosed eating disorder and would like to work with a skilled clinical hypnotist, please advise your therapist of your choice and the hypnotist of the diagnosis and encourage them to collaborate. When I am collaborating with a therapist, I am careful to assure them that I will allow them to direct the focus of our hypnosis practice to achieve the objectives they think most beneficial. I also feel free to present them with the information I have gathered from working with the client and even my interpretation of that information, but they are the ones with the training and experience that has earned them the license to practice mental health.

Joseph A. Onesta

Chapter Seven: Stage Two

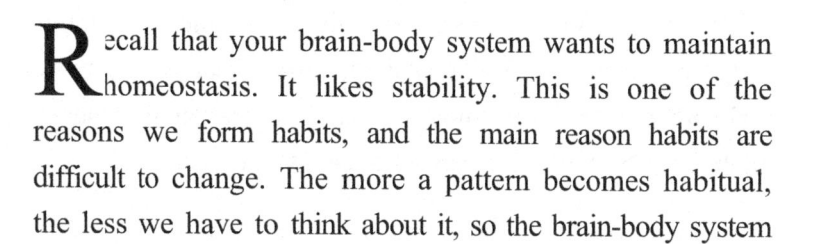

Recall that your brain-body system wants to maintain homeostasis. It likes stability. This is one of the reasons we form habits, and the main reason habits are difficult to change. The more a pattern becomes habitual, the less we have to think about it, so the brain-body system creates habits (patterns of thought, behavior, and reactions) by *averaging* out our experiences and perceptions.

Those habits or patterns can be changed, but the brain-body needs a sufficient reason for making the change. In other words, when you go on a temporary diet, your brain-body doesn't believe it is a change but a temporary condition to which it must temporarily adapt. When those temporary diets are sustained over a long period of time or are habitually conducted, the brain-body settles on the condition of semi-starvation and resets the metabolism lower so that when the diet is finished, the weight comes back very quickly.

In the Onesta Process, we focus on gradually changing the averages so that the brain-body accepts a new normal that we can also live with. Consider, for a moment, your average natural fast. Let's say that you commonly snack just before going to bed at 11:00 p.m. and you eat just after waking up at 7:00 a.m. Your average natural fast is 8 hours. Your brain-body expects to eat after eight hours. At the appointed time, your stomach may already be preparing for digestion, your liver may stop producing glucose, and your pancreas might already have started kicking out more insulin.

When you don't eat breakfast at the usual time, your brain-body might begin to insist on eating, partly because your body is already prepared for eating. You've broken a pattern. Hunger might become naggingly persistent and even urgent.

When we gradually change the averages, the body learns to adapt to new patterns without the shock of a temporary change. If we maintain those changes long enough, the body will simply accept those changes as a new normal, making them a natural part of life.

Look at your average natural fast. At this point, we want to consider that average a minimum, whatever it is. If your average is 12 hours, *we* want to extend the average by an hour or two each week either by adding fasting time before bed or after waking. When you take your last caloric bite for the day, calculate the time the following day after which you will eat. If your snack ends at 9 p.m. and your average natural fast is 12 hours, tell yourself you will eat sometime after 10 a.m.

Notice that I did not suggest you tell yourself that you will eat *at* 10 a.m. but *sometime after* 10 a.m. It's a self-hypnosis hack to give fair warning to your brain-body not to expect to eat until after that hour. You may still feel hungry, but you'll have more ability to simply put off eating until the time you said.

As long as you are setting 12 hours up as a minimum, your daily natural fast will be more than that, and so will the average. We want to increase the natural fast by an hour or even two per week until we reach the minimum of 16 hours.

Additionally, I also suggest that when you set the ending time for the natural fast, you also plan what you will eat: "Sometime after 10 a.m., I'll have bacon and eggs." You can always change your mind, but if you plan the next meal, you won't be frantically scrounging for food or reaching for just anything that may be available at the moment. Remember, you will likely feel hungry then and (at least at first) will have to battle a bit of hunger until the averages are up to goal.

It's a good time to let you know that breakfast, when you break your natural fast, can happen anytime. It doesn't have to be in the morning. A morning breakfast is not the most important meal of the day, no matter what the breakfast cereal manufacturers say. Continue tracking your natural fast so you can average it weekly and track your progress.

By the time your average natural fast is at least 16 hours, your daily natural fast might sometimes be upwards of 18 hours. I know it sounds like a lot. I remember having to fast 10 hours for bloodwork, and I found that really hard. For most people, 16 hours may actually be a long time to fast. That is why we do this gradually. Every week, extending the natural fast a bit more until we get there.

We are doing this for two reasons. First, we are giving the body time to use the glucose we consumed the day before and potentially have time to begin accessing glycogen. The liver loves doing this. Second, we are building up our tolerance for not eating so that when we attempt our first real, therapeutic intermittent fast, it will be easier to do.

Identifying and Reducing Carbohydrates

Now take out your photo album of what you ate over the last week. Look carefully at each plate and determine what percentage of the plate, by visual volume, consists of carbohydrates.

If you didn't take pictures of your food, go back and repeat Stage One. You are not really ready for Stage Two, and your benefit from this process will be significantly limited if you don't follow the plan. Taking pictures is not only a practical act; it's a psychological one. We need to change your mind as well as your body. You need to *see* your food differently. We are changing perceptions as well as plate composition.

If you did follow directions, congrats. You win. Let's go on.

We have three purposes for identifying and reducing carbohydrates. With reduced carbohydrates, both your hunger and cravings will eventually fade. Because your blood glucose levels are more steady, your carbohydrate hunger is minimal.

Carbohydrate cravings are also part of a phenomenon called the cephalic insulin response. When your stomach, pancreas, and liver aren't getting the normal carbohydrate levels they expect, they signal to the brain to look for them and the brain creates those cravings. This phenomenon is one of the primary reasons I encourage my clients to avoid artificial and non-nutritive sweeteners.

When someone drinks a diet soda, the taste buds note that they are consuming something sweet. The taste buds send a message to the brain registering sweetness. The brain, thinking sweet means sugar, sends a message to the stomach, the pancreas and the liver to expect glucose. The stomach creates digestive juices, the liver stops creating glucose out of glycogen and the pancreas secretes insulin in preparation.

But it was a diet soda. There is no sugar there. When the stomach and the pancreas register that the sugar has not arrived, they signal to the brain, asking, "Where is the sugar?" While in your conscious mind you know there was never any sugar in the soda, the taste buds signaling the brain didn't know that. Now the brain begins to search for things that will create the sugar that the stomach and pancreas are demanding. The person may feel hungry or crave sweets or carbohydrates to supply the expected dose of glucose.

The second reason for reducing carbohydrates is important for the healing of the body. With the reduction in available glucose, the cells in your body have more opportunity to use stored glucose. Insulin-resistant cells will eventually take down the barriers they have set up when the deluge of glucose stops. Your body will begin to access glycogen or stored glucose more readily, and if we keep up the reductions in carbohydrates, your liver will begin to more readily convert fat into energy. You will be burning fat, even while you sleep!

So, take a hard look at those pictures and identify the carbohydrates on the plate. Anything that contains sugar is a carbohydrate. Because of the high sugar content, fruit is considered a carbohydrate. Forget the phrase "fruit and vegetables." While they are both plant-based, they are far from similar.

All foods made from grains such as wheat, oats, corn, rye, barley, rice, and even quinoa are carbohydrates. All vegetables that grow below ground, like potatoes and carrots, are carbohydrates. It may be surprising that beans and legumes, while containing protein, also carry enough carbohydrates to be classified as carbohydrates and not protein.

Vegetarians and vegans beware. Negotiating the carbohydrate and protein balance is tricky for you. Some people who are vegetarians allow themselves to eat eggs, dairy, and seafood. The process is easier for them. But when I am working with a vegetarian or vegan who has only vegetable sources of protein, we have to resign ourselves to compromises that slow down the process, limit the achievement of goals, or rely heavily on processed foods, which come with complications of their own.

I was a vegetarian for about 20 years. I remember a nutritionist showing me 400 calories of beans and comparing it to 400 calories of lean meat. Notice that she focused on calories and not protein to carbohydrate ratios. Considering that plant protein is less accessible to the body at 17% absorption compared to animal protein at 30% absorption, one has to consume a lot more protein from vegetable sources than from animal sources. The irony, of course, is that vegetable sources, also containing carbohydrates, leave people feeling hungrier sooner after eating.

Don't be discouraged. Most people eat mostly carbohydrates. But you now understand that those carbohydrates are raising your blood sugar and stimulating the production of insulin, which increases your insulin resistance.

Our first big change is to consider those portions of carbohydrates and, from this point forward, cut them in half. A burger and fries become an open-faced sandwich, and you offer half your fries to someone else. Feel free to fill up your plate with protein and above-ground vegetables. No need to limit yourself to lean meat, either—your body needs the fat, and eating fat does not make you fat. Eat butter, not margarine. Use heavy cream instead of skim milk.

Because of our fear of fat, we have rendered most vegetable dishes bland and tasteless, as if the only way to eat vegetables is steamed. Feel free to experiment with veggies: sauté, roast, and stir fry using saturated fats like coconut oil, bacon fat, butter, lard, or duck or chicken fat. Explore sauces, seasonings, and dressings. Just avoid commercial dressings that are generally filled with sugars and seed oils. Recipes by people who follow the ketogenic diet are all over the internet. Go on a vegetable adventure.

Another way of amending your plate is to add a soup course. Good quality bone broth, preferably homemade, forms a great base for a hearty stew. A cup of soup is a great way of introducing quality collagen, fat, and whatever else you choose. Just avoid starchy vegetables, grains, and grain-based noodles. Mung bean sprouts, lentil sprouts, any kind of leafy greens, green beans, broccoli, cauliflower, brussel sprouts, snow peas, beaten eggs, and left-over meats make wonderful soups. Puree them with a bit of heavy cream or coconut milk for a creamier texture.

If you still feel hungry at the end of a meal, have ready a bit of cheese (the harder the better), olives, nuts, or full-fat yogurt with a few berries. Fat makes us feel satisfied longer. I personally like to finish my meal with salad, and often that salad contains olives, cheese, and pumpkin or sunflower seeds. My mother used to say that vinegar helps in digestion. Of course, she never bought commercially bottled dressings.

Continue plating everything you eat. Take pictures of every plate. And always eat intentionally, without distractions. When you sit down to eat, mentally tell your brain-body that you are about to eat. You are training it to not assume when you will eat so that it learns not to trigger those automatic digestive functions until it needs them. I know it sounds fantastic, almost unbelievable, but most people are unaware of the power of their own minds and intentions.

It is fine to drink while you eat but sipping a beverage between each bite is inadvisable. While most habitual dieters do not overeat in general, sipping a beverage can lead many to do so without realizing it. In a later chapter, we will explore the subject of satiety, that is, feeling satisfied. Because liquid simply passes through the system, the feeling of satisfaction may not last as long when every bite is washed down with a sip of something. Drink water before your meal and after it, but control how much you drink during the meal.

Consider replacing your snacks entirely with high-fat foods that will stimulate satiety. Cheese, olives, hard-boiled eggs, and nuts are good choices.

Doing this gradually is important because drastic changes are less sustainable. We will proceed through the stages at a pace you choose and one that you find comfortable. We need to have reached a 16-hour natural fast before progressing to Stage Five.

If you have chosen to track blood sugar, you should continue to measure your blood glucose daily, just prior to your first bite or sip of the day. Note your daily readings. Average them out at the end of each week and note the averages.

About 50% of my clients are comfortable going on to stage three after a week at stage two. The other half want another week to get used to the reduced carbs. No matter what we decide, the natural fast increases weekly. We never go beyond two weeks at this stage because we've only just begun and need to get moving for some results.

Continue tracking and noting your natural fast and averaging it out weekly. Weigh yourself and check your waist size weekly, ideally at the same time of day, most commonly when you wake up in the morning. Note the numbers, but if there is no change at this point, don't let that discourage you. You are doing well.

Chapter Eight: Food

"All things are permitted," but not all things are beneficial.

1 Corinthians 10:23 (New Revised Standard Version)

Processed and Manufactured Food

From the peeling of fruit to the discovery of fire, human beings have been processing food. When we butcher meat, when we grind grain, when we chop vegetables, when we season, cook, and preserve food, we are processing it.

Processing is not necessarily bad, but there is a real difference between the kind of processing we do in our kitchens and what is done in factories to produce the food we find pre-packaged at the supermarket.

Let's follow the food manufacturing process from the beginning to see how much of our food supply is far from "natural" or even "healthy," no matter how the package is labeled. In fact, you should discount any product labeled as healthy or natural because, in product labeling, those terms do not mean what most people would think they mean.

Industrial agriculture and animal husbandry practices are based on profitability. The storybook images of farms growing a variety of fresh vegetables and with barnyards housing a variety of livestock are far from reality. Miles of land dedicated to single commodity crops such as corn, wheat, and soy are the reality. Farms cover our land producing commodities, while huge warehouses of animals are fed on grains that they would never eat in the wild, grown in soil that has been so stripped of its natural nutrients that petroleum-based chemical fertilizers, pesticides, and herbicides have to be used to maintain profitable production.

The grains, the foundation of our agriculture, have been genetically modified to make them resistant to pests and resistant to herbicides that are sprayed to control weeds. Vegetables have been genetically modified to be bigger, have a longer shelf life, and better withstand the rigors of being shipped around the world. While the Food and Drug Administration (FDA) has declared these foods safe for human consumption, there is little hard science backing up that claim, especially in the long term. The very basis of our food industry is unnatural.

The FDA has also designed nutritional recommendations that conveniently coincide with industrial food culture. We are told to eat up to 60% of our caloric intake in grains and cereals. It's mighty convenient that we have those in abundance due to government subsidies. The power of food industry lobbies cannot be overstated, and the policies held in the supposed best interest of the people come into serious doubt.

The vast majority of our food supply has been rendered unnatural. Debates and exposés over the past decades have revealed the potential of a food system that is at best less healthy, and at worst toxic. Indeed, many of the biggest causes of death and disease in our society are directly related to metabolic disease.

The purpose of this chapter is to present a summary of what I see as important aspects of those debates that we can directly control ourselves. We always have a choice of what we do and do not eat. While I believe that changing the system is a worthy objective, that change won't come in time for many of us. The current trends toward convenience, packaged food, meal plan subscriptions, and supposed miracle-nutrition super-food concoctions, including the move toward plant-based foods, indicate a significant barrier to that change.

What you adopt and embrace from this chapter is entirely up to you. I urge you to do your research and investigate your sources of information. You can start with the recommended reading list at the end of this book.

The Whole Grain Myth

We were told that up to 60% of our diet should come from "healthy" whole grains. Even if we leave out the genetic modification of grains, the difference between whole grains and refined grains is minimal. Whole grains are ground and pulverized just like refined grains. The only difference is they leave the fiber in the whole grains. While this may slow down digestion a bit, blood glucose still spikes with whole grains and causes a corresponding insulin response.

The standard dietary recommendations were based on the faulty science presented by Ancel Keys in his heart health hypothesis, in which he vilified saturated animal fat as increasing the risk of cardiovascular disease. While inaccurate, his findings were widely accepted. Despite the protests of other reputable scientists with sound evidence to support their objections, Keys' hypothesis was eventually adopted as an official recommendation not only by the FDA but also by the medical and nutritional professions, and even spread to other countries.

The Big Fat Lie

Those seed oils touted as healthy alternatives to animal fat are chemically extracted. In simple terms, they use chemicals to separate the components of grains such as corn, canola, rapeseed, sunflower, or soybeans to find the oil. (You can't squeeze corn and get corn oil out.) I'll take butter and lard over margarine and shortening or seed oils every time. Seed oils oxidize easily when heated and the negative health consequences of heated and oxidized vegetable oils are more than worrisome.

Seed oils have been linked with many modern diseases including inflammation of the bowels, an imbalance of microbiome, digestive system inflammation, and the weakening of intestinal walls, not to mention susceptibility to food allergies and digestive diseases like Crohn's disease and irritable bowel syndrome.

One mitigating factor is if oils are labeled as expeller-extracted, cold-pressed, or extra virgin. Generally, this means that what you are apparently buying is the easy-to-get (not chemically extracted) versions of these oils. Unlike corn, they squeeze olives or avocados, and oil does come out.

Good vegetable sources of oil are pure, extra virgin olive oil. Olive oil has a low-temperature smoke point and is not the best for frying. It oxidizes too easily and is better used as a condiment, in salad dressings, or drizzled atop roasted vegetables just before serving. Avocado oil is better for cooking as it has a higher smoke point and carries no real flavor of its own. Coconut oil is a vegetable source of saturated fat, but it does have a flavor that may affect the taste of your dishes.

Many vital nutrients like vitamins A, D, E, and K are fat-soluble, meaning they need fat to be absorbed by the body. A low-fat diet, especially one that relies on manufactured seed oils rather than saturated fat, may be a source of deficiency in these vitamins.

The concern about fat in the diet is hotly debated

because we have become a society concerned about cholesterol, and thus have become a society of people taking cholesterol-lowering medications. I point out that the value of these medications is questionable. The cholesterol argument grew out of Keys' hypothesis and subsequent studies indicate that not only was his hypothesis wrong, but it was also harmful. There are a number of factors emerging from science that indicate that the use of cholesterol as an indicator of potential cardiovascular risk is not as accurate as are triglycerides.

Of course, many people believe that eating fat makes people fat because a gram of fat has twice the calories of a gram of protein or a gram of carbohydrates. But we know that the creation of body fat requires two things, insulin and excess glucose. Glucose stimulates the pancreas to create insulin and excess glucose is converted into body fat. When glucose is minimized, the body accesses fat as a fuel source, converting it into ketones. The entire body, including the brain, loves ketones.

The science indicating that saturated fat causes cardiovascular disease is based on the assumption that Ancel Keys was right. He was demonstrably wrong, but the establishment finds it difficult to admit the error of buying into Keys' theory.

Our society has turned our food culture into a chemical experiment. Read the ingredient list of just about any product from the inner aisles of the supermarket, and you find something that is more chemical concoction than natural food. It looks like food. We like the taste and even crave it, but does the body recognize it as food the way it recognizes and uses real, wholesome food?

The Fiber Fib?

I'm not going to make a big deal about this, but it is important to know that the body has no real mandate to consume carbohydrates. We like them. We love sweet things. But the desire for high carbohydrate food is one part evolutionary and nine parts cultivated.

In evolutionary history, when tribes of people wandered about looking for things to eat, particularly looking for things to kill and eat, they sometimes stumbled on things like berries and grains. They ate them and liked them. Archeological artifacts called *querns* (grinding stones) show us that they even processed them, though the processing was far cruder than today's refining processes. Of course, the supplies were limited and the occasional indulgence in a berry patch or apple tree served to fatten them up a bit for the winter when times were leaner.

Carbohydrates didn't become staples until people settled into agriculture, and in many locations during the feudal world, the game—that is, animals—were the property of the rich landowners. Poor folks had to glean from the remnants of the crops and make do with what they could find and occasionally poach.

While I personally do not subscribe to a carnivore diet— that is, a diet that consists solely of animal products—the notion that the body somehow needs carbohydrates is false. The idea that carbohydrates are necessary is based on the understanding that glucose is a necessary fuel for the body.

It's true that the body uses glucose more than it does fat, but in modern times, the balance has been upset. Your body may be using some fat, especially when it needs to absorb nutrients. Evidence suggests that even obese people are always burning fat to some degree, but in an environment with an overabundance of carbohydrates, that usage is minimized.

Carbohydrates are not necessary. Recall that I pointed out that upwards of 70% of animal protein is actually converted into glucose. Only about 30% is absorbed as protein. We don't need additional carbohydrates. We like them. We enjoy them. But we don't need them.

If we eat a diet that centers on protein and we enjoy a healthy amount of above-ground vegetables, we will have access to all of the nutrition we need as well as sufficient fiber to feed our microbiome, the bacteria in our gut.

Humans don't actually digest fiber, the microbiome does. Beans are a magical fruit that makes us toot because the microbiome excretes gas as it digests the fiber. In other words, you are farting the farts of digestive track bacteria.

On more than one occasion, clients and colleagues have asked me about the concept of *net carbs* in the ketogenic diet. The theory goes that if you are following a strict ketogenic diet, consuming fewer than 30 grams of carbohydrates a day, you can use the concept of net carbs to stay on track. One considers the carbohydrate content of a particular food and subtracts the fiber content from the carb count. A serving that contains 12 grams of carbohydrate and 3 grams of fiber, is believed to average out to 9 grams of carbohydrate per serving.

Keep in mind that they are intentionally eating fewer than 30 grams of carbohydrates per day. That means they are counting all carbohydrates, including the ones in vegetables. If you want to embrace a ketogenic diet, go for it—but you'll need a kitchen scale and some math skills.

In the Onesta Process, we do not count anything, and the notion of net carbs is not important to us. I confess, when I am making a purchasing decision about a processed ingredient I want to use in a recipe, I look at the carbohydrate content and it feels better to consider the net carbs. But know that the use of a processed ingredient, such as an alternative flour, is in fact, a compromise away from complete control of a whole, real food eating plan.

Real, Natural Food

Real food is food that can be found in nature in the form that is used in the kitchen. Flour, by definition, is not a real food unless the ingredient list includes only the unrefined grain of the flour—in other words a bag of wheat seeds. Everything else is an intentional compromise that I make consciously. So when I am making tortillas for soft tacos, for example, I know the macros for the recipe I use, and the ability to eat the tortilla takes precedence over whatever carbohydrates the recipe indicates. The keto version may not taste exactly the same but better serves my long-term objectives.

Natural food, in my definition, is organic: free of pesticides, herbicides, and chemical fertilizers. It was cultivated from non-GMO seeds. The meat I consume comes from animals that were treated humanely and were allowed to graze the way they would naturally.

The truth is, there are lots of compromises along the way. I can't afford to eat like this all the time, but I am conscious of and intentionally make the compromises I see as necessary to be able to live and eat the best way I can within my budget. I do not simply throw up my hands and say, "There is nothing I can do about it, so to heck with it, I'll eat whatever." Each compromise is a conscious one.

One of my biggest complaints about the ketogenic diet is that it has become a fad money maker for food processors. There is a wide variety of highly processed, highly refined, chemically derived food products that claim to be "keto-friendly." People who don't know what they are doing are deceived by that label into thinking that those products are healthy and will help them control their weight. Think again, please.

All "keto-friendly" means is that they have added fiber to facilitate the net carb calculation and may have chosen some alternative ingredients, such as non-nutritive or artificial sweeteners, that don't carry as many carbohydrates as the traditional ones. You might think frozen pizza with a cauliflower crust is low in carbohydrates but read the ingredients and the nutrition labels and you'll find out differently. The same is true for keto cookies, keto ice cream, keto cakes, keto breakfast cereals, and almost any other manufactured food product labeled keto. In order to not be fooled by labels, you need to learn how to read the labels. And if that means bringing a magnifying glass to the supermarket, do it. I never buy a food product without reading the labels.

Ingredient Lists

In the United States, food manufacturers are required to list the ingredients included in a food product in descending order by weight. The first ingredient is, by weight, the biggest ingredient.

If there are ingredients that you don't recognize as a whole food, it's probably a chemical derivative. The definition of "natural flavors" is ambiguous enough to be suspect.

Some ingredients are blatantly chemicals. If you don't know what it is, why would you want to eat it? Given that many of these chemicals are emulsifiers or flavor enhancers, it is advisable to actually look them up. Xanthan gum, for example, is an emulsifier derived from corn. It helps replace some of the role of gluten as does psyllium husk, a fiber used as a laxative. Flavor enhancers like monosodium glutamate or yeast extract cause side effects for some people. Know what you are eating.

Any ingredient ending in "-ose" is likely a sugar or sweetener. We'll address non-nutritive sweeteners a little later in the chapter. Sugar is addictive and was likely used to replace the fat in manufactured foods because fat is a natural flavor enhancer. Microdoses of sugar add up. This alone may be a reason to avoid choosing a manufactured product, considering that sugar and sugar derivatives may appear several times in the ingredient list.

Any ingredient that follows the phrase, "Contains 2% or less of" refers to each ingredient listed, not the cumulative total of the following ingredients.

If I am totally honest with you, any food product that lists a seed oil, often soybean or canola oil, gets put back on the shelf unless I have no choice, which is almost never. I always have a choice.

Nutrition Information Labels

Please ignore the last column on food nutrition labels, which indicates the recommended daily amount or percentages. Those calculations are based on the standard dietary guidelines, which are inherently flawed.

If you are an experienced dieter—that is, a calorie counter—you already know about the serving size snag. The serving size is smaller than what most people might consume in a single serving. The good news is that we can skip the corresponding calorie count. Calories don't count, so we won't bother. We are, however, concerned about the carbohydrate content and the sugar content. While the carbohydrate content includes sugar, we must understand that sugar is half sucrose and half fructose. While sucrose is converted into glucose and used throughout the body, fructose is processed only in the liver. Since fructose is not converted into blood glucose, it does not spike blood sugar like sucrose and carbohydrates.

That fact makes fructose sound promising but there is a snag. Since fructose is processed only in the liver, we should be concerned about fatiguing it with too much fructose. The liver is critical to our healing process. While fructose does not spike blood sugar, it does trigger increased insulin through the cephalic insulin response. While it is important to control blood glucose to avoid the physical deterioration caused by chronically high blood sugar levels, an important aspect of reversing diabetes is reversing insulin resistance. Hyperinsulinemia, elevated insulin blood levels, cultivates insulin resistance.

We are reducing our carbohydrate intake because it reduces blood glucose and consequently reduces the need for insulin. Elevated insulin is as much of a problem as elevated blood glucose.

Therefore, when looking at the nutritional information, we need to consider what effect consumption of the product will have on our insulin levels via spiked blood sugar. If the carbohydrate content of a single serving seems high, the food is not worth eating, no matter how much your mouth is watering.

If you choose to count carbs and embrace a strict ketogenic diet, keep that choice as a maintenance goal. There are too many people who cannot sustain a ketogenic lifestyle and end up going back to the way they were before trying. If you follow our process, you will achieve ketosis and you will be in a better position to make a choice about a strict ketogenic lifestyle.

Sugar

Sugar is a carbohydrate. It is also a dose-dependent hepatotoxin. That means sugar in tiny amounts can be safely handled by the liver, but it is toxic in more than moderate amounts. Unfortunately, sugar in various chemical forms is in nearly every processed food available in a supermarket. If you are wondering exactly how much is safe, we can assume that most people are consuming toxic amounts of sugar on a daily basis. This taxes the liver and contributes to fatty liver disease and non-alcoholic cirrhosis of the liver. Refined table sugar is about fifty percent fructose, which can only be processed and eliminated by the liver, thus making the sugar itself even more toxic.

Alcohol

Most people are aware of the carbohydrates in beer, but while we are on the subject of food, we should address alcohol in general. Remember that this process doesn't forbid anything, but not everything is beneficial. There is a condition called non-alcohol-related cirrhosis of the liver that comes from consuming too much sugar and carbohydrates. Your doctor may have used the words "fatty liver," which is a kind of precursor to cirrhosis. As fat accumulates in and around the liver, the liver begins to suffer. Chronic fatty liver disease can lead to cirrhosis, just like too much alcohol can.

It stands to reason, then, that drinking alcohol to excess will affect your ability to achieve results from this process. It should also be obvious that any alcohol at all, just like any sugar, would represent at least a slowing down of the effectiveness of the process. It is a choice now, and forever a choice.

I've never said you can't have something, no matter what it might be, but we have to weigh the consequences of indulging in any food or beverage that distracts us from our journey to wellness. What seems absolutely harmless to most people may represent a formidable obstacle toward our ultimate success.

Avoid alcohol as much as you can. Remember that we are not forbidding it but consider the cost of what seems like a small, momentary pleasure.

You don't have to drink alcohol to drink socially. I used to drink socially when I was young and went to clubs. I never really liked the taste of alcohol, but that didn't mean not getting drunk. I used to drink a cocktail called Long Island Iced Tea, which just tasted like sweet tea. A couple of those as a young man put me in some embarrassing situations, one of them quite dangerous. There comes a point when growing up is more important than being one of the guys.

I decided to avoid alcohol, but I still drink socially. I ask the bartender to give me seltzer water with a wedge of lime. It looks like a cocktail. I can act silly without alcohol and nobody knows the difference. The only catch (I learned this the hard way) was that I couldn't let friends buy me a drink. I'm willing to stand a round as much as the next guy, but on more than one occasion, when a playful friend thought getting me drunk might be fun, I found myself looking for a place to discreetly abandon the glass or bottle. My true friends got the idea sooner or later, and while it was tedious always being the designated driver, at least I still had fun.

Once you reach your goal, a small glass of wine with a meal now and then or an occasional beer might be choices you make, but you need to make those choices, and only you are responsible for the consequences. Until you reach your goal—that is, until your new body weight has become your new normal—just consider avoiding alcohol as part of your healing process.

If avoiding alcohol represents a problem or even just a hurdle for you, consider working with a qualified clinical hypnotherapist. You don't have to be an alcoholic to need this kind of help. In fact, if you recognize an active addiction, get the help you need from a qualified professional drug and alcohol counselor.

Chapter Nine: Stage Three

The reason we continue to take pictures of our food through several stages is to allow our perception of the number of carbohydrates we are consuming to change. What originally looked like normal consumption of carbohydrates will seem excessive in a few weeks' time. That is a milestone to look for.

At the end of stage three is commonly the last point where we continue taking pictures of our food. Some clients who have trouble making cuts or still have trouble managing their carbohydrate decisions will need to continue taking pictures of their plates in stage four. Others will find the picture-taking a kind of accountability they continue to value.

Take a moment and compare your stage one photographs with the more recent ones. Did you really cut the portions in half? Were there times you fudged a little? You wouldn't be the first to try that. Did you notice that your snacks were almost 100% carbohydrates? In stage two, a plate with six cookies might become three, but the plate is still 100% carbohydrates. In stage three, if you are continuing to snack, you should think about snacks that can replace carbohydrates with either protein or fat. I am assuming that you are snacking only within your eating window, the time you have to eat before your next natural fast begins.

Consider, for example, a hard-boiled egg, a small handful of nuts, a few olives, or some cheese as a snack. If you want crunch, pork rinds are an option, but be careful of the seasonings applied. You can look for keto cracker recipes online and start experimenting. Pickles can add crunch, just avoid the ones made with sugar. You can dehydrate certain vegetables to become chip-like, but avoid the underground or starchy ones.

It's best if you give up snacking all together and eat only during meals. Snacking represents one of the areas where some clients demand compromise. If you insist on snacking between meals within your window, make wise choices.

The next steps are comparatively easy, but only if you've been following the process faithfully. Cutting corners slows down the process and potentially limits results. One of the key advantages of working with a trained hypnotist and coach is that they can help you with the changes you find challenging or with understanding the consequences of compromising on specific aspects of the process.

Now, consider the most recent photos. Identify the remaining carbohydrates on the plate and, once again, cut them in half. Throughout this stage, you should be consuming only about 25% of the carbohydrates you were consuming in stage one.

You can always add a bit more protein to your plate, and veggies that grow above ground are usually less starchy and have fewer carbohydrates. Consider green beans and snow peas as better choices than other beans or peas because we also consume the shell. Explore salads as a side dish but avoid commercially produced salad dressings, even the ones that promise to be low-calorie. We aren't concerned about calories, and commercial dressings are often loaded with sugars, sweeteners, and seed oils.

When you finish a meal, you should be satisfied—not stuffed, not overly full, but satisfied. In other words, you do not feel hungry anymore. You could continue to eat, but the feeling of urgency is not there.

If you still feel hungry at the end of your meal, have seconds. My clients usually raise their eyebrows in shock when I say that but honestly, in the years I've been doing this, I've had very few clients for whom overeating was a problem.

As you proceed through this stage, it commonly becomes clear that one or more forms of carbohydrates simply become ***not worth eating***. When an ear of sweet corn becomes a quarter ear, hardly more than a tablespoon or two, some clients decide that the corn isn't worth the bother. Others, however, might eliminate another carbohydrate, say a scoop of mashed potatoes, in order to keep the corn.

I have one client who swore she could not eat eggs without a piece of bread. She firmly stood her ground on that point. You and I both know that her statement was not a truth but a perception. When she drew that line in the sand, I asked her to search for keto bread recipes. She agreed and finally found one that worked for her; but even as a hypnotist, getting her to erase that line in the sand was a battle not worth waging.

I am indicating the kinds of internal negotiations clients go through during this phase. I spent a lot of time and money trying every form of low-carb and keto pasta recipe I could find and even tried to invent several of my own, all to disappointing results. Eventually, I was ready to accept that pasta, the way I used to eat it, was simply not worth eating at all. But the struggle was real, and I had to work my way through it. Believe it or not, I don't miss pasta.

My husband and I went to visit my godmother, whom I hadn't seen since lockdown. She made a big Italian Sunday dinner with spaghetti, meatballs, salad, and chocolate cake. As we sat down at the table my husband whispered, "You are going to eat this. Your godmother made it and you are going to eat it."

Of course, I ate it. I ate reasonably moderate portions. I worried that eating that meal would kindle my pasta cravings, but it didn't. That meal probably had more carbohydrates in it than I had eaten cumulatively in six months. It was good. I didn't hate it but I didn't like it as much as I used to. I was fine getting back on track.

When your mind decides that a certain food isn't worth eating anymore, it becomes very easy to resist the temptation to eat it, even when there aren't many alternatives. By the end of this stage, if any cravings for carbohydrates remain, they will be psychological or emotional urges, which you now have other ways of addressing.

I used to love corn on the cob. It was at this stage in my own process that I determined that corn as a side dish was no longer worth eating. I haven't bought corn since. But one day, I was in a restaurant with friends. I ordered a chicken fajita salad without chips, rice, or beans. When it arrived at the table, it came laced with corn kernels. Perhaps I hadn't read the description as well as I should have. I suppose I could have sent the salad back but I'm not a jerk and I didn't want to wait for them to remake the salad. I also could have opted to take it home instead of eating, feigning not being hungry. Instead, I ate the salad and made a mental note to read menus more carefully. I didn't fall into corn cravings. I couldn't say that I even tasted the corn. It certainly didn't add much more than a filler to the salad bowl. In my mind, sweet corn is still just not worth eating.

As I mentioned earlier, I've had very few clients who demonstrably overeat. In fact, most of them are obviously undereating. They aren't getting enough nutrition, notably protein, out of their meals. They focus on portion control and eat just enough to push away from the table, but then they pepper the moments with tiny, nearly inconsequential snacks between meals to tide themselves over until the next meal. They do this almost to the point of absurdity. One client during stage two took a picture of five jellybeans on a plate. Seriously, five jellybeans.

Keep in mind that if you don't eat enough, your body will go into conservation mode and you will not lose weight. Semi or even complete starvation for an extended period of time changes the metabolism and makes it both difficult to lose weight and very easy to regain it.

Because perpetual yo-yo dieters are likely to constantly feel a bit hungry, let's talk about what it means to eat until you feel satisfied. Let's start with a definition. Feeling satisfied simply means you do not feel hungry. If we are satisfied, we could always eat a bit more. If we do, we become full. If we eat beyond that point, we begin to regret it, finally admitting we have eaten too much.

The problem with chronic dieters is that the space between being satisfied but not overstuffed disappears. Psychologically, they may feel "hungry" until they are overstuffed. Or they may have accepted that feeling hungry all the time is normal.

You have been reducing your carbs, so carbohydrate hunger should be a diminishing problem. Hopefully, you've been filling your plate with protein and vegetables because we don't want you to simply eat less. Eat less was the mantra of the old paradigm. We want to eat until we are satisfied. That means having seconds of things that are not carbohydrates and eating until, upon reflection, feelings of hunger are not present.

Let's do a little mind-hack. Take a moment to close your eyes and ask yourself, on a scale of 0 to 10, with 0 being overstuffed, and 10 being ravenous, how hungry do you feel right now? We never want to feel ravenous, and we never want to feel overstuffed. If ravenous is 10, a sustained feeling of hunger somewhere between 7 and 9 might be a good time to admit that you don't feel satisfied. If your number ranges between 3 and 5, that's what satisfaction feels like. Let's say 1 to 2 is full. Note that it isn't hunger until 7. Even at 7 to 8, we could probably still wait until the next meal.

Of course, there is room in your stomach to have a little snack, but you aren't really hungry. When we eat a meal and we eat until we are satisfied, we psychologically tell ourselves, "I'm not hungry anymore. I'll eat again at the next meal. No need to snack in between. I'm good until then."

When your hunger pangs between meals, either you didn't eat until you were satisfied or the feeling of hunger is one of the phony stimulations that make us feel hungry, as was illustrated in a previous chapter.

When we get into therapeutic intermittent fasting, you will have to postpone real feelings of hunger, at least at the beginning of the process. So do yourself a favor and identify what satisfaction—not being full or overstuffed—feels like.

Heed the warning. No matter how much you believe in calories, they do not count. If you aren't eating enough food, your weight loss will slow down and even stop. Because your body believes the situation is temporary, your liver will keep your blood glucose levels higher than you like, and breaking that cycle may cause you to regain weight.

If your average natural fast has reached a minimum of 16 hours, just keep to that pattern until we reach stage five. When your natural fast averages between 16 and 18 hours, you have time to eat at least two, possibly three full meals during your eating window (the hours in the day when you are not engaging in a routine natural fast).

If you have not reached a minimum of 16 hours, continue extending your natural fast by an hour or two each week until you do. Remain in this stage until you reach that threshold. From this stage forward, we will maintain at least an average of 16 hours of natural fast throughout the process.

Now let's take on insulin resistance more directly.

Insulin resistance is when the cells of the body are so full of glucose that they resist taking on more. By reducing the carbohydrates in our diet, we have also reduced the need for insulin in our bloodstream. Lower levels of insulin are necessary to begin reversing insulin resistance.

Though it is an oversimplification of the process, we can begin to reverse insulin resistance by increasing the use of the glucose already in our cells. This is done through increased activity or extending the time between meals (or both). When cells use the energy they have stored, they will become more willing to accept glucose replenishment from the blood, whether it comes from what we eat or is manufactured by our liver from stored glycogen or fat.

We can encourage the cells of the body to use the glucose they have in one of two ways. The easy but slow way is to just wait. Eventually, your cells will use the glucose they have and be willing to take on more. The better way is to force the cells to use their glucose more quickly.

Do some form of gentle exercise that moves muscles, increases our breathing, and perhaps raises our heart rate just a little. Do it every day. We might walk the dog, clean the kitchen, do the laundry, or vacuum the carpet. Playing dance music during household chores actually causes you to move a little faster.

Of course, if you enjoy working out, then you should work out. Go ahead, pump iron. Take gym classes like water aerobics, spin, or Zumba. Get on the treadmill or the elliptical. It doesn't matter; just move. Just make sure you are doing it or something like it every day.

Anyone who has ever used electronic exercise equipment that estimates the number of calories burned during a workout knows that exercise, especially intensive exercise, is useless. Half an hour on a treadmill typically burns fewer calories than one consumes in a piece of toast.

Science tells us that when we exercise intensely but irregularly, the body goes into a kind of emergency mode similar to semi-starvation. It becomes conservative with energy and creates hunger to replenish what was used. More often than not, the resulting hunger can replenish the energy used in just a few bites, but usually we consume more than a few bites. Depending on what we eat, our blood glucose levels rise in the process. We increase insulin and actually *gain* body fat. How about that! Exercise can make you fat! We might temporarily benefit from extra cardiovascular activity, but ultimately all we get from intensive exercise is hunger.

We want to begin gradually increasing our activity levels. We want to encourage the body to get used to needing and using more fuel on a regular, normal, basis. If done appropriately, you won't overeat. After all, your body has plenty of fuel stored in your fat cells.

Many of my clients start with a pedometer app on their phone. Your phone is something you carry with you throughout the day. Just set up the pedometer to track your daily steps. Forget the artificial goals that the apps suggest. Ten thousand steps may well be out of range for many people at this point. Keep it simple. Every day, just walk a few more steps than the day before. If you like data, track the averages—because average is what the brain-body considers normal. Then on a daily basis, go a few more than average. As the average increases, add a few more to that.

There may be days when you are exceptionally active. We would not count those days in our average simply because they are not part of the normal or regular activity levels. If you take your time and increase your average activity levels gradually, your brain-body will adjust its idea of what is normal for you.

Eventually, you'll begin to notice that on days that you are less active than what your brain-body thinks is normal, you will have excess energy and you'll have more get-up-and-go because your brain-body wants to get up and go. When that happens, it's time to look for more exertive activities that you enjoy.

Most people hate going to the gym and working out, but if you enjoy it, go ahead. But don't limit your activity to three times a week. Go every day and alter your workouts. If you can't go every day, find something else to do on days you can't go. Activity levels are not exercise sessions, they are consistent and averaged over time.

The important thing is that whatever you choose to do, you enjoy it enough to look forward to doing it again tomorrow. To find what you would enjoy doing, consider sampling the free sessions offered by many businesses that offer classes such as yoga, Tai Chi, martial arts, or dance lessons.

You should enjoy it enough to do it frequently, and it should inspire you to get better at it. It doesn't have to be just one thing. You might go bowling once a week, walk the dog every day, go to dance classes once a week, martial arts or yoga two or three times a week. Consistency and gentle increases over time are the keys to raising average activity levels and avoiding exhaustive, punishing exercise.

Most people are inclined to be involved in activities that are prosocial. That means that you see the same people over and over again. You don't have to become besties to experience the extra motivation created by prosocial activities. You might see the same people at the gym if you go at consistent times. If you are in a class, you'll get to know others who attend that same class. Don't be afraid to introduce yourself and try to remember the names of the people you meet.

In my book, *Deleting Diabetes: I Did it. You Can, Too,* I recounted an event that demonstrated my own progress. Just before Christmas, I was in an automobile accident. I was unharmed but my car was totaled. I tried shopping for a car, but the ones I could afford, I didn't want. The ones I wanted, I couldn't afford—at least without incurring significant debt. So, I took the bus to work.

Pittsburgh is a city in the foothills of the Appalachian Mountains. We don't have mountains, but we have hills. Lots of them. In fact, communities actually built municipal steps to help people take shortcuts when they walk. With the exception of certain limited areas, any real walk involves plenty of up and downhill stretches.

My walk to the bus originally took me down a set of municipal steps plus another 15 minutes to the bus stop. On the way home, it took longer because it was all uphill. When I started taking the bus, coming up nearly 100 municipal steps was a challenge that required several stops to catch my breath.

Over time, I noticed that I could more easily push through the uphill climbs, stopping fewer times. Then I could make it all the way home in one go. But that's not the best part.

My commute required a bus transfer in downtown Pittsburgh. One day, as my first bus inched through traffic up to my stop, I saw my connecting bus round the corner and stop. If I missed that connection, I'd be waiting another 30 or 40 minutes. Without thinking, I bounded off my first bus and sprinted to the second. I caught it. As I found my seat on the bus, I realized that I was not out of breath despite having run a bit more than an entire city block. The real shocker, however, was that I had run at all and I had done it without thinking. I was in my late 50s at the time, and I hadn't run anywhere for any reason for probably 20 years. I've even missed connecting flights because I refused to run through an airport.

I want you to see how small changes really do add up and make a real difference. I am not a kid anymore, but there is no reason I can't become increasingly fit, active, and confident.

Please take it easy. Some people want to jump into the deep end of the pool before they learn to swim. They try to make far more drastic cuts than the process suggests. I implore you not to do so. You may at this point discover that there are carbs you can very nearly eliminate, but please do not cut out all carbs. Please do not subject yourself to extensive fasts at this point. We will get to longer fasts soon, but not yet. We are not cutting calories, nor are we starving ourselves. I know it's natural to want rapid changes, but slow and steady is the only way to reset our default settings. Jumping into the deep end only increases the effort and decreases the likelihood of success.

During this stage:

- Consume less than 25% of the carbs you consumed in stage one. Eliminate the carbs that are just not worth eating.

- Try to avoid snacking between meals or replace your snacks with better snacking choices.

- Increase your natural fast weekly until your minimum is 16 hours a day on average. If you have already reached that threshold, maintain it through stages three and four.

- Weigh and measure your waist circumference weekly and note the changes.

- Increase your activity levels gradually. The more muscles you use, the more glucose you burn and the more you are reversing insulin resistance. Just don't overdo it. Keep it gentle and progressive.

- Generally, clients remain in stage three two to three weeks.

Chapter Ten: Checking In

Some people lose weight quickly and others do not. In my experience, nothing about my weight seemed to change at first, but I have already confessed that I think I was experiencing a bit of body dysmorphia, seeing myself as fat when I had lost a considerable amount of weight. Recall that I hadn't been weighing myself because my primary concern was my diabetes.

In the time I've been working with clients, I've seen all sorts of patterns emerge. Some lose weight right away. Others seem to stay the same and then experience a precipitous drop in weight. Still others seem to lose one or two pounds at a time. Hopefully you have been tracking your weekly progress.

In my work with clients, I make sure to track their

progress session by session. At this point in the process, I will often plot my clients' progress on a chart so they can see the trends. We take time to discuss the nature of the changes in both body and mind.

In every session, I listen to what they say and take notes when I notice shifts in their thinking. Most people don't notice these shifts, but because I'm hyper-aware of them as part of my job, I notice them in myself as well.

The first time I realized that I fit into a seat on an airplane I marveled. I used to desperately hope for a window or aisle seat simply because I could overflow the seat either toward the window or into the aisle. On a recent trip, I noticed that my seating posture had changed as well. Throughout my life, I've sat crossed armed and legs together on airplanes.

On this trip, I noticed that my posture was what some people describe as man-spreading. I was comfortable in the seat. My knees were pretty far apart, at least for an airplane seat, and my elbows were situated on the armrests. I was in an aisle seat so I had a bit more room but the row was full and the person sitting in the middle seat had his arms crossed, the way I used to. He was a pretty big guy and I conversationally mentioned he should allow himself to be comfortable while trying to give him room. He didn't take me up on that.

There is a lot of time to think about things on an airplane, and I considered the change I had noticed. It occurred to me that I no longer felt the need to make myself smaller. I was no longer sensitive about my size or how it might affect other people. I wasn't being rude. I wasn't even being greedy about the space. I was just comfortable in my own space.

I sometimes notice my clients walking differently as they lose weight. They slouch less. They relax more. Their stride is more fluid and comfortable. They have more spring in their steps. They seem more confident.

They sit and talk differently, too. Instead of sinking into the chair, they might sit forward. Their voice has more energy to it. Not a nervous energy that comes from anxiety but rather a paced energy that comes with excitement and a brighter outlook. Believe it or not, sometimes I can see it in their eyes and even in their complexion. They may have actual improvements in their skin. Rashes and acne clear up and they look less tired, more alive.

Did you know that skin tags are a sign of metabolic disease? Yours will go away as your body heals from metabolic disease. Your blood pressure may drop, and skin conditions will lessen and even disappear. You'll think more clearly, be more attentive, and more alert. You'll even sleep better.

Of course, my clients and I would have been working on confidence, self-acceptance, and authenticity as part of our coaching and hypnosis sessions. Part of me knows that these changes aren't my doing. My job is to help them do it themselves. I can't do it for them, but I can work with them. Yet I marvel at the changes, the very ones we have been working on and that makes me feel wonderful. And I know that the improvements they see even at this point give them permission to better occupy the space of their lives, the way I occupied the space in my airline seat.

These changes are as much mental and emotional, even spiritual, as they are physical. At this point, I'm thinking about you and your journey and I'm feeling a little sad that I don't know you and can't observe any of your changes. I'd love to point them out to you because I know that unless you are a very reflective person with some training in hypnotherapy, you probably don't see them yourself. Take another full body picture the way you did in stage one. Don't compare the two, not yet. Wait. Save them for the end. It will be worth it.

You probably have improved more than you realize, but I can't be there to point out those improvements. If things don't seem to be going according to plan, consider the following obstacles that might be getting in the way of progress. These are not meant to judge you but to help you troubleshoot your experience, if necessary.

- There may be hidden sugars or carbohydrates in your diet. Remember that consuming carbohydrates always stimulates insulin and even tiny amounts can stop gluconeogenesis, that is when the liver uses glycogen to create glucose.
- Are you still consuming processed or manufactured

foods? These often conceal sugar under various names. Even condiments and things like salad dressings often have sugars or sugar substitutes. Beware of supposedly *keto-friendly* processed foods. Also, processed and manufactured foods deliver chemical cocktails to our digestive system that may be slowing down your progress.

- Perhaps you haven't cut carbs as much as you think you have. People tend to eat in patterns meaning they often have similar meals. Consider going through your photographs and comparing similar plates. How is the carb cutting going?

- Continue to take pictures of your food and reduce carbohydrates even more. You will eventually cut out some carbohydrates as completely not worth eating, but others you may keep for one reason or another.

- Are you eating fruit and have you forgotten that fruit is a carbohydrate? Remember fruit is not only a carbohydrate, but also high in sugar and fructose. It's going to raise your blood glucose and tax your liver. The best fruits to consume are small amounts of berries. Pairing the berries with natural, unsweetened, full-fat greek yogurt or homemade unsweetened whipped cream are amazing treats.

We really cannot measure the level of healing and change that is taking place inside your body. If you are measuring your blood glucose, you should have seen some lowering of the average fasting glucose levels. Your pancreas is able to function in a more normal fashion. Your liver, provided you have mostly abstained from sugar, fructose, and alcohol, is in the process of healing and honing its function. Actually, it has already begun to regenerate.

If you found some of the bullet points above challenging, you are not alone. Often when I am working with clients, they express reservations about their ability to accept some of the changes we will make on a permanent basis.

One client dubbed herself a "carboholic" and resisted cutting her consumption of many carbohydrates. She was using her self-imposed label to justify her resistance to the kinds of changes we needed to make. She insisted that she hated to cook, could not cook delicious food, and preferred to rely heavily on restaurant takeout and frozen dinners. Every session, she would laughingly admit to the occasions she didn't follow the plan, and those occasions made all the difference. Sbe seemed to refuse to make better eating choices. "It came with fries, so I ate them. After all, I paid for them."

After three or four sessions, I chose to prorate a refund to her and send her on her way. I don't like firing clients. I wish I could help everyone, but that isn't the case. People like her think that hypnosis is magic or mind control. It just doesn't work that way, and even the most talented hypnotist cannot make a person go against their will.

I only accept weight loss clients who need to lose at least a third of their body weight. I really would rather spend my time with clients who embrace what we are doing. My carboholic wasn't willing to change. I can't compete with that.

Some clients read ahead of the program. They read through the whole book before beginning their journey. When they see what we are doing, they determine they can't or won't do it. They become overwhelmed by the prospect of where we are going and decide not to go there. They are like the carboholic who drew that line in the sand. That's why I encourage my readers to take it step by step. The changes we make today make the ones we will make tomorrow easier. No one thinks they can do this until they do it.

My experience and those of my clients tell me that tastes eventually change. The sweets they once craved, for example, have become too sweet. Fries may smell and taste of rancid oil. One client admitted to biting into a hamburger bun and spitting it out because to him, it felt like a cotton ball in his mouth. Becoming more sensitive to sweet things is pretty universal, but a cotton ball bun was a unique description.

Others realize that their sensitivity to wheat gluten becomes more noticeable, even if they consume even small amounts of wheat. Gluten is known to have a negative impact on the microbiome. Sensitivity to gluten is not as severe as Crohn's disease, but after going a long time without eating gluten, they are more aware of the upset it causes in their digestive system.

By now, you are probably not craving carbohydrates the way you once did. I'm not suggesting that the food you once enjoyed won't stimulate positive memories. I experience this every time I go to a festival where funnel cakes are being sold. But I can and do avoid funnel cakes without difficulty because I know that if I eat some, I won't enjoy it the way I once did—because I have changed.

Indeed, there will be changes that we live with for the rest of our lives but eliminating all carbohydrates completely and forever was never part of the program. This process is not about never eating carbs again. Rather, it's about being in touch with your body and maintaining a healthy relationship with the food you choose to eat.

If you have established any degree of regularity, by now your hunger patterns have changed, especially if you have begun crushing cravings and controlling your emotional eating. You'll notice that if you regularly eat at a certain time of day, that is when you are feeling hungry. If you have been eating intentionally, you can manage even those feelings of hunger by simply telling yourself, in a self-hypnotic way, when you plan to eat. The mind-hack works.

It is important that we eat well during our eating window. We should avoid eating untold quantities of just anything that happens to be lying around. Some people think that as long as they are starving themselves the rest of the time, they can have whatever they want during their eating window. Nothing could be further from the truth. If I haven't made this clear enough yet, you can't have your cake and eat it too.

But, did you catch the flawed and debilitating thinking? Reread the last paragraph and underline the words *starving themselves*. We are not starving ourselves. We are not fasting to reduce calories. We are giving our bodies time to heal by increasing our natural fast. When we eat, we need to eat nutritious, real food that helps our bodies heal themselves.

One of the reasons we put our snacks onto plates to begin with was to be aware of mindless eating from packages. If you eat a handful of nuts every time you pass the bag, you'll eat more nuts than you are aware of. But who ever said that you couldn't put as many nuts on the plate as you wanted? True, we cut the carbs in half and then in half again. Not nuts.

You can avoid snacking all together by eating each scheduled meal until you are satisfied. At the end of the meal, use the mind-hack of mentally reminding your unconscious mind when you plan to eat again. In the meantime, if hunger pangs seek to distract you—like nagging kids in the backseat of the car asking, "Are we there yet?"—the answer is simple: "No, not yet, but soon."

You are not depriving yourself of anything. Instead, you are making better choices. Eating well means eating good, fresh, whole, nutritious food that will deliver the nutrients and energy the body needs without triggering too much insulin production. Believe me when I say, you will come to crave and prefer that kind of food over the sh*t available in most fast-food restaurants.

I attend and present at several hypnosis conferences a year. I am fully aware that the available restaurants are likely to serve food that doesn't appeal to me or that is inconsistent with my lifestyle. I will ask the hotel for a refrigerator if they have them, visit a grocery store, and buy things I want to eat. At conferences, we often eat meals together, and on those occasions, I do my best but often have to compromise my standards. That's life.

Let's keep in mind what we are doing. We are changing our lives.

Chapter Eleven: Stage Four

———⚜———

I want to congratulate you. If you've come this far, your commitment to taking ownership and responsibility for your own health and the quality of your life is established. Well done!

What changes have you noticed in yourself? Have you lost weight? Has your waistline changed? Have your average fasting blood glucose levels lowered? If so, celebrate the changes, but keep going. We aren't done yet. If not, keep going. We aren't done yet.

From this point forward, we will maintain an average of 16 to 18 hours of natural fast. We want this to become normal for us. An 8-hour eating window that corresponds to a 16-hour natural fast is plenty of time to have three, well-appointed meals if that is your choice. Many clients prefer two meals a day. Some of them add a small snack in the middle. If that is the way they choose to run their non-fasting days, so be it.

Once the brain-body mechanism grows accustomed to this schedule, you will not normally experience hunger during your natural fasting time. You will also be less likely to reach for snacks during that eating window as long as your meals are centered on protein and contain sufficient fat.

Your job, from this point forward, is to maintain at least an average 16 hour natural fast. That will likely be true for you for the rest of your life.

We will also continue to reduce carbohydrates, but from this point forward, no specific requirements will be made. You do not need to continue taking photographs of your plates as long as carbohydrates represent less than 20% of what you normally consumed in Stage One. If you find it helpful to continue taking the photographs, go ahead, but it's not required.

From here on out, your reduction in carbohydrates will change focus (keeping in mind that the more carbohydrates you cut, the better your results will be). We can eliminate a significant number of the remaining carbohydrates because *they simply are not worth eating*.

A client once remarked something along these lines: "When the kids were home, I made them a sandwich with some chips or fries for lunch. I sometimes pinched one or two for myself. Now that they are back in school, I don't even think about chips or fries. I don't make them for dinner anymore, and I don't even bother having them in the house."

The very idea of food that is not worth eating is probably new to most people, but it is one of the landmarks we see on our journey through the process. Something worth eating is something that will not only quell our feeling of hunger but will also nourish our bodies and help our systems continue their healing and restoration processes. Anything that goes counter to those purposes is not worth eating.

Even so, there will be carbs you decide not to cut out entirely. Instead, you will limit the frequency with which you choose to eat them. People may indulge in a piece of fried chicken or breaded shrimp on rare occasions. They might satisfy their curiosity with a forkful of a dessert or some apparently starchy food they've never tried before.

There will come a time when you realize that carbohydrates in most meals are just a cheap and easy way to fill the plate. If you go to your favorite family restaurant and order a burger and fries and eliminate the carbs, for example, you are left with a dry hamburger patty, a slice of tomato, some token amount of lettuce, and a pickle slice. Is that worth the price of the dinner you are paying for? There is a reason why restaurants that offer healthy alternatives like a side of broccoli or a side salad make those replacement choices so small, tasteless, and uninviting. It's cheaper to fill your plate with bread and potatoes.

Therapeutic Intermittent Fasting

I've mentioned before that therapeutic intermittent fasting is different from extending the natural fast. In the Onesta Process, a therapeutic intermittent fast is at least 24 hours.

There are people in the world who simply extend their natural fast on a daily basis, perhaps eating one meal a day. This eating plan is known by the acronym: OMAD. People who regularly practice OMAD are often just increasing their natural fast to about 23 hours. There is nothing truly *intermittent* about this practice. I fear that many ill-informed people have adopted this form of semi-starvation or reduced-calorie diet as a lifestyle, thinking they are doing something therapeutic.

If they are eating sufficiently for their body to function properly and they are getting all of the nutrition they need, I have no cause to complain, but I find it difficult to believe they are doing that in a single meal. That said, the only objection that remains to OMAD is when they call this practice *intermittent* fasting. Again, there is nothing intermittent about practicing OMAD.

Fasting simply means not eating for a time. Intermittent means that there is no sense of regularity established. What makes intermittent fasting *therapeutic* is the reason we are doing it. Many people fast to reduce calories. In their minds, they fast to lose weight. Losing weight is not our intention.

Naturally, we will consume fewer calories on fasting days, but calorie reduction isn't the point. Some people try to weigh themselves after an intermittent fast hoping to see weight loss, only to be disappointed when the weight comes back a day or two later.

In preparation for therapeutic intermittent fasting, we have been extending our natural fast. You may think this has something to do with eating less. It does not. By extending our natural fast, we have been reminding the body to rely on gluconeogenesis, the creation of glucose from stored energy. We have been gradually pushing the body in the direction of performing gluconeogenesis—earlier and more consistently.

Because of our previous high-carbohydrate diet, our bodies have grown unaccustomed to needing to produce glucose from energy stores. We have been working up to this moment, training our bodies, preparing them for this very moment.

Your first 24-hour fast is like the first race after your training period. Or if you are less sports-oriented, how about your first recital after practicing the piano? You might be nervous. You might doubt your ability to make it. You can and will make it, I promise.

When we choose to engage in a fast of 24 hours or longer, we are putting the body into the position of utilizing glycogen stores that may not have been depleted in years. When a healthy, fit person goes to bed, glycogen should be sufficient to get them through until morning. That's what they are for. However, in a person with insulin resistance who has chronically high levels of blood glucose, it may take longer to deplete the liver's glycogen stores.

Because we have been reducing our carbohydrate intake, our bodies require less insulin. As a result, insulin resistance naturally begins to decrease. When we increase our activity levels, remember, we are not burning calories but rather using the glucose in our muscle cells. When they need more glucose, they will lessen their resistance.

When we fast for 24 hours or more, the body will use up its ready glucose. The liver will begin gluconeogenesis to maintain a steady supply of blood glucose. Once glycogen stores are depleted, the liver will begin to access fat, eventually creating the alternative fuel called *ketones* in a process called *ketosis*. This may or may not happen as a result of this first fast. We'll talk a bit more about ketosis in the next chapter.

I normally suggest that my clients do two 24-hour fasts each week until our next meeting or until we progress to stage five. For the sake of ease, I recommend that those days **not** be sequential, simply because I want my client to see each fast as unique and complete.

Pick a busy day. The busier you are, the easier it will be to avoid eating. However, if you are a stress eater, make sure you set aside time for some simple relaxation activities, such as breathing exercises, short walks, or side-line projects for a change of pace.

Include your natural fast in the 24-hour period. It seems unnecessary to state this, but you are already fasting regularly for at least 16 hours. All we are doing is extending the fast by a few more hours.

Start your fast after a meal and go from meal to meal. You can go from breakfast to breakfast, lunch to lunch, or dinner to dinner. Note the time you finish eating and consciously announce to your brain-body, "I'll eat again tomorrow sometime after (pick a time). I'll be fine until then."

Plan your next meal. You can always change your mind, but you don't want to be frantically looking for something to eat when you reach your goal. Build that meal around protein and fat. Make it a no-carb meal. Meat and above ground vegetables are good choices. This meal is going to "break" your fast, so there is nothing wrong with breakfast foods like eggs and bacon.

Handle hunger pangs and cravings, the way you have been, and remind your brain and body when you will eat again. "I will eat again sometime tomorrow after (time)."

Prepare an escape plan. No one goes into battle without at least having some sort of escape plan. This first battle is more psychological than physical, no matter how hungry you think you are. Knowing there is an escape plan helps many people stand their ground. I suggest having some good, wholesome bone broth ready to heat.

Normally, bone broth would be considered something that might break a fast. It is not something we would normally drink during a fast. However, bone broth is better than breaking the fast entirely by eating. If the bone broth is good quality, it contains both fat and collagen and is flavorful. After all, it's soup without the solids.

Set your escape plan in motion if your mind becomes fixated on eating, you stare at the clock watching the minutes tick by, or you find yourself laying down, clutching your stomach in hunger. Look at the clock. Tell yourself you can have your broth in an hour, and then get up and get busy. The hour may pass unnoticed. If it does, extend the promise another hour. If not, and you can't get away from the frantic thoughts of needing to eat, heat up the broth and mindfully sip it.

Enough people use their escape plan the first time around, but once we make it to 24 hours, we know we can do it. Future 24-hour fasts become easier and more routine.

Again, do two 24-hour fasts per week until you are ready to move on to stage five.

Always take your prescribed medications when fasting, but check to see if the medication you are taking controls blood glucose or presents the potential of hypoglycemia. If your medications make this precaution, call your doctor before attempting this and future therapeutic fasts. Your doctor should give you guidelines for reducing or eliminating medications during a therapeutic fast.

Proper hydration is always important, but even more so during therapeutic fasting periods. This is an opportunity for your body to cleanse itself. During longer periods of fasting, your body speeds up a process called autophagy. In the process of autophagy, the body begins to eliminate and recycle damaged and redundant cell material, literally metabolizing it in the process. The body is always cleansing itself, but during longer periods of fasting, the process is heightened.

The liver and the kidneys are central to the function of cleansing and the consumption of clean, filtered water greatly facilitates the process.

If you have eliminated most processed foods, your intake of salt has likely been significantly reduced. Processed and manufactured foods are often high in salt, and when we shift our diet to more natural, real, whole foods, we may actually need to add salt. Choose a high-quality salt that provides some mineral support. High-grade sea salt or the now common pink Himalayan salt are better choices than common table salt.

Many people confuse hunger with thirst. It is extremely important to stay hydrated while you fast. Good, filtered water is the best, but there is nothing fast-breaking about black, unsweetened coffee or teas, including herbal teas, either hot or cold. Avoid diet drinks sweetened with either artificial or non-nutritive sweeteners, as these are still likely to trigger an insulin response.

Keep in mind that we are reducing carbohydrates because they trigger high levels of insulin, not because of their calories. Elevated insulin levels cultivate insulin resistance, so reducing our need for insulin is critical for reversing the problem.

Chapter Twelve: Opposition, Ketosis, and Autophagy

Well Meaning Opposition

The moment people notice changes in your behavior they become curious about what you are doing, especially when they see that you are losing weight. Everyone is looking for fast and easy solutions to weight loss, and their curiosity will peak.

I've learned from experience not to flippantly tell people what I am doing. If I use words like low-carb or intermittent fasting, they roll their eyes because they see these practices as fad diets, and most of them will stop listening. Some will voice objections such as, "I tried that for a while. It didn't work," or "The weight just came back." Unless you are willing to engage in a lengthy conversation about why what you are doing is different from the fad diet they tried, just keep your mouth shut. If they genuinely want to know more, refer them to this book. If they are diabetic, refer them to my book *Life Without Diabetes*.

We all come with the baggage of the diet and exercise marketing world. We've all been trained to think that eating less and exercising more are the keys to fitness and that if we are fat and out of shape, it's because we are lazy gluttons. If you've read this far, you now know better than this—but the world doesn't. The world is still looking for magic pills, superfoods, and meal replacement shakes.

Even if you do engage in the discussion, very few people are willing to really listen. I have very good friends, people that I dearly love, who have completely written off my achievement as something that won't work or, at least, won't work *for them*. They themselves are morbidly obese and extremely diabetic. You'd think they really want to know how I did it, but they don't. These are the same people with whom all I have done over the last 20 years is eat. Going out to eat is what we do.

Unfortunately, going out to eat with them comes with inherent conflicts.

They eat late. I am usually finished eating by 7:00 p.m. I'm an early riser and often in bed by nine. When we meet, we usually meet for dinner, and we meet at seven or later. I can alter my schedule to accommodate their schedule and have done so often enough. Also, I know that a single divergence in my natural fast will balance out. After all, we want to focus on the average. But I don't like to eat late. I don't sleep as well if I go to bed with a full stomach. Changing my hours might mean giving up a good night's sleep.

I prefer to be with them and not eat but, they cajole me. They seem to take offense if I choose not to eat with them. I've had to stand my ground more than once and I have learned to simply tell them that I am not hungry, that I have already eaten. Still, they push me to at least get *something* or offer me tastes of their food.

I think they do this because they feel awkward eating in front of me. I have on occasion ordered something and simply did not eat it, either taking it home for a different meal, perhaps to throw it away or just leaving it on the table. I hate doing that.

I've taken to assuring them that if I were hungry, I would eat. I really do want them to know that I joined the party because I wanted to be with them. After all, eating is just an excuse for being together, isn't it? I joined them because I wanted to enjoy their company and if I don't feel like eating at the moment, I free to not eat.

If I happen to be fasting, even during my natural fast, I never tell anyone that I am fasting, ever. I tell them I'm not hungry. It's not a lie. Even if I feel a bit hungry, I know that I'm not really hungry. The hunger I feel may be triggered by the food, the company, the atmosphere, or something else. I now choose when to agree with hunger pangs and when to ignore them, and I am perfectly comfortable doing so.

Needing to alter eating schedules at home can be a complicated matter. My own partner would accuse me of starving myself when I would fix dinner and not eat it because I was on a fast. There were times when I just didn't feel like cooking, and another argument would try to surface when we ordered out or went to a restaurant and I simply did not order anything for myself. I'd try to assert that I was just not hungry, but that excuse wouldn't always work. My partner and I had to have serious and direct conversations about what I was doing and why.

When children are involved, the process becomes even more complex because we may have mixed emotions about what we are feeding our families. I don't have children, but have had clients who have experienced a broad range of problems.

Most families, especially those with teenagers, don't eat together these days, something I consider very sad. The upside of this is that issues about why mommy or daddy isn't eating dinner have been rare.

More common are children who are exceptionally picky eaters, usually in favor of processed foods. What begins as a quirk of a childish palate quickly grows into a problem of adolescence and can be a significant limitation in adulthood. I've had parents bring their picky children to me to expand their palate. Hypnosis can help, but they have to want to expand their palate, and few kids really do. I confess that I do not often work with children and feel slightly guilty when I refer parents to other practitioners.

I'll gladly help an adult expand their palate, but it is as much instruction and coaching as it is hypnosis. And it is a long process of unlearning. With children, who are often unwilling, the process to get them to be willing is daunting.

Many parents overfeed their children food that is patently unhealthy. The percentage of carbohydrates children consume in this country is setting them up for future metabolic disease. If a partner insists on high-carbohydrate meals, we can rationalize that they are adults and can make their own decisions. But with kids, we are in charge of what they eat.

Of course, we can simply just let them eat what they have been eating. When problems arise, we can deal with them then. However, what good parent would be willing to intentionally do that? Some get frustrated, give up, and hope for the best.

Very gradually reducing the carbohydrates on a child's plate is excruciating, especially when the child whines and gets moody. Smaller portions of carbohydrates, incorporating more protein and fat into the meals, limiting sweets, and teaching children that treats are not food takes time, patience, and perseverance. It also requires navigating the traffic jam of other people, such as grandparents, who want to indulge them. It's virtually impossible to ignore when, after soccer practice, the parent providing snacks has chosen some pre-packaged "healthy" snack loaded with carbohydrates and sugar for the team.

Here are some tips to keep your sanity while navigating this process:

- If you can't control what they eat in school or at extracurricular activities without being one of *those* parents, don't. Just let it go.

- Stop filling your pantry and freezer with convenient, processed, or manufactured food products.

- As often as possible, eat at least one meal a day together as a family. Control that meal. Make it delicious. Ban cell phones, television, and any other distractions during the meal.

- Gradually change the macronutrient ratios on their plates. Smaller portions of carbohydrates, and larger portions of protein and tasty vegetables.

- If a child refuses to eat something, let them not eat it, but explain that there is no replacement for it and there won't be any snacks later. Snacks should be considered treats, not regular food. You control the snacks in your house and when they are available. If they go hungry after a meal, their body will manufacture the glucose they need and there is always tomorrow. The alternative is to have ready non-carbohydrate replacements such as cheese, olives, pickles, salad, or limited amounts of processed meats like pepperoni, salami, or luncheon meats.

- Save dessert for one day a week and make it exceptionally good. Consider homemade whipped cream (heavy cream and a bit of vanilla) or Greek yogurt with berries (frozen then thawed, no sugar needed). Make it pretty, in parfait bowls or goblets. The internet offers a plethora of recipes for keto or low-carb desserts.

- Make vegetables tasty and exciting. Again, the internet has wonderful recipes that either come low-carb or can easily be made low-carb. Adding color, fat, and seasoning can make a vegetable dish more enticing.

- Prepare and clean up after that meal together, even with little children. Teach kids how to cook things that are within their abilities. A five-year-old is capable of helping you stack the dishwasher, even if you have to rearrange some things.

- Model reading labels for your children. If they ask for something from the grocery store, patiently understand they are responding to the package, advertisements, and what they see their peers eating. Limit choices and still provide treats now and then.

- Reduce the convenience aspect of eating. You don't need a snack or sugary drink every time you fill your gas tank. You don't need to grab anything off the shelves immediately near a check-out register. You don't have to zip through a drive-through window to feed your family. If you do, your priorities may need some attention.

- Make treats rare. Stopping for ice cream should be a special occasion. Cake is for birthdays. Cookies and candy are not food.

- Above all, play the long-haul game. Small changes pleasantly made over a long period of time, really do add up.

We have talked about gluconeogenesis before. This is when your liver begins producing glucose from stored energy sources. Ketosis happens when your body knows you mean business. Your body can make two different kinds of fuel out of fat. It can make glucose, as in gluconeogenesis. And it can make ketones, as in ketosis. In fact, to a large extent, your body is always using a little fat, even if you have been following a low-fat diet.

While the transition from gluconeogenesis to ketosis can be a bit uncomfortable for some (see Keto Flu below), once the transition takes place, most people feel great, have greater clarity of thought, experience very little hunger, have more energy, and even sleep better. Some, however, report bad breath.

Prolonged strong ketosis appears to have been associated with the occurrence of kidney stones in a small percentage of people, mostly children. I had a client who is a nurse bring up this issue. I have not found studies that conclusively indicate that ketosis *caused* kidney stones. The two conditions happened together, but there was no cause-and-effect relationship demonstrated.

I am frequently in and out of ketosis and I have opted to take a cranberry supplement, as cranberries have been shown to have preventative properties regarding kidney stones. If you are worried about kidney stones, take a cranberry supplement. In any case, the supplement will not harm you, but drinking the actual juice will prevent or kick you out of ketosis because of the sugar content. If you are prone to kidney stones, you may want to consult your doctor regarding the use of a cranberry supplement.

The Ketogenic Diet

Anytime there is a strange word to identify something, there is a bit of mystery about it. Understanding what the ketogenic diet is will help you distinguish between a low-carbohydrate diet and a ketogenic diet. Keto has become for many just another fad diet, resulting in a plethora of questionable processed food products and gimmicks.

Simply put, a ketogenic diet is designed to consume so

few carbohydrates that the body switches to making ketones as a primary source of fuel.

A ketogenic diet consists of extremely reduced carbohydrates, usually fewer than 20 to 30 grams of *net* carbs daily. These carbs are usually found in fresh vegetables and rarely, if ever, in grains. You may choose to count carbohydrates or "calculate the macros" as many ketogenic dieters do, but that is a matter of your own decision.

In its simplest form, it comes down to measuring portions and calculating how many grams of net carbohydrates you are consuming. Take a step or two up and you are looking at what percentage of your diet is dedicated to each macronutrient.

Biohacking

Many people on the ketogenic diet engage in biohacking. Minimally, they test to see if they have remained in ketosis. Others strive to move deeper and deeper into ketosis. Some engage in experiments to see how they respond to different foods, particularly *resistant starch*. Resistant starch is a carbohydrate that takes longer to digest and ends up fermenting in the large intestine instead of being digested in the small intestine.

Whole grain bread is made from flour that has been finely ground. There is no reason to believe that whole grain bread is more resistant to digestion than white bread. The indigestible fiber certainly takes up some room, but the rest of the kernel is fully digested.

Some believe that starches, such as rice, can be converted into resistant starch by freezing and reheating. There are internet influencers who engage in such experiments as part of their video offerings. The biohacking experiments are interesting to watch, but I want to raise a few cautions that responsible influencers doing biohacking should also point out.

Resistant starch experiments, while seeming to indicate a result, speak more of the condition of the individual than of the food being tested. The experiment is insufficient evidence to make a wider claim. The results of the experiment should not be taken as evidence that the same thing will work for you to the extent that it worked for the experimenter.

Resistant starch biohackers haven't changed their minds about certain foods. Unlike participants in the Onesta Process, they still look longingly at those foods even if they are successfully avoiding them. Many ketogenic biohackers are frustrated to some degree about the limited role of carbohydrates in their diet. They are psychologically living in an environment of dietary restriction. We, on the other hand, have gone beyond the point of wanting our cake and eating it too.

The purpose of many ketogenic dieters is weight loss, not healing the body of metabolic disease. They may test their blood glucose and ketone levels as part of the experiment, but their interest lies in the ketones, not the glucose. For them, the danger of glucose lies in the reduction of ketosis.

Ultimately, they may well be eating a lot of processed,

refined, and manufactured food products. Indeed, many of them promote products that I call Keto Krap—for example, keto cookies, cakes, ice cream, and breakfast cereals. All of it is highly processed, often containing unhealthy chemical ingredients. Just because the macros seem to add up, often depending highly on the dubious notion of net carbs (adding fiber to apparently counteract the carbohydrate content), doesn't mean the food is healthy or good. It certainly is far from natural.

A short-term biohacking experiment on resistant starch only indicates that they can eat a certain food *if* it is prepared in a certain way. In my mind, that is more restrictive than allowing my body to heal from metabolic disease by being aware of what I am eating. Having reached my goal, I have enough wiggle room to eat something outside of my new normal. But the important thing is, I don't want to. When I'm sitting around with friends at a birthday party, I do not ruminate on my inability to have cake. I don't want the cake, and it is not a matter of exercising willpower. I know I won't like it.

How will I know if I am in ketosis?

It is possible that you have already been in ketosis to some degree. Many people are in ketosis after a 24-hour fast. The discomfort some might experience, known as keto flu, may have been chalked up to the discomfort of the fast.

There are two ways to test the level of ketones. You can purchase inexpensive test strips. You hold the test strip, placing the coated tip in your stream of urine. If the coated tip changes color at all, you are in ketosis to some measurable degree. These should be sufficient while you are on the program. If you choose to follow a strict ketogenic diet, you may consider buying an electronic device, similar to a blood glucose meter, that measures ketones.

Keto Flu

So far, no one knows why some people suffer flu-like symptoms when adjusting to a ketogenic diet. They are generally temporary, lasting at most a day or so. The reported symptoms are fatigue, constipation, feeling foggy or unclear, irritability, nausea, or headache. Keto flu most often happens once and never again.

Fat Adaptation

As you surf the keto world, you will hear the phrase "fat adapted." The existence of ketones in the blood, urine, or breath does not mean your body is fat adapted. Your body can use both glucose and ketones for fuel. Often, particularly when following a low-carbohydrate diet, the body is actually using both kinds of energy. When the balance tilts firmly toward ketones as a primary fuel, and the brain adjusts to using ketones rather than glucose, you are said to be fat adapted.

Ketoacidosis

Some people are afraid of ketosis because they have heard of a serious medical condition called ketoacidosis. The condition is real but also rare and happens in the ***absence*** of insulin. In order for insulin to be absent, your pancreas has to stop working. If you are eating meat and vegetables, your pancreas will be producing insulin. Recall that upwards of 70% of the protein in meat is converted into glucose. Glucose means insulin is present. Unless you suffer from Type 1 diabetes, a condition in which the pancreas does not produce insulin, you need not overly concern yourself about ketoacidosis.

Autophagy

The word literally means *self-consuming*. Autophagy happens continuously, to a minor degree. When your body recognizes a cell that no longer serves its purpose, it will recycle it. The healthier you are, the more efficiently and seamlessly this happens.

When you stop poisoning your body with unnatural chemicals like those found in processed foods, your body can focus its attention on honing autophagy. The busier your organs are eliminating toxic chemicals, the less they are involved in autophagic processes. But when we engage in therapeutic intermittent fasting, while eliminating those chemical toxins, the body is freer to remove malfunctioning cells and expend energy on producing new, healthy tissue.

Autophagy increases the more the body experiences starvation. Let's call it what it is: When we fast beyond the reserves of glycogen in the body, unless we eat something, the body perceives a certain amount of starvation and shifts its fuel source to maintain equilibrium, or homeostasis.

This is the primary reason we stress the word intermittent in the fasting process. We don't want the body to perceive famine, which can result in an adjustment of metabolic rate. In other words, starvation diets, such as reduced calorie programs, often lower our metabolism and thus make it all the easier for us to overeat (and regain weight) when the temporary diet ends.

When we fast for longer periods of time, but not long enough for the body to perceive famine, we allow the body to use energy stores as fuel while focusing on cleansing—that is, autophagy. The meals we consume after a period of therapeutic intermittent fasting should center on proper nutrition, which can come fully from quality protein and fat.

Chapter Thirteen: Stage Five

At this point, I don't have to remind you that avoiding carbohydrates only helps our progress and allows our bodies to heal more. By now, there are some carbohydrates that you have eliminated entirely as simply not worth eating. If, when you look at your plate, you automatically consider the ratio of carbohydrates, you are where you should be. If there are carbohydrates that are still tempting, those you think you can't live without, I suggest you challenge that assumption.

If fries or potato chips plague your thoughts, I suggest going without them completely for several weeks. Look for replacements from the keto recipe community. (They're really good at that!) After three or four weeks without that powerfully tempting carbohydrate, mindfully taste it again.

You may well discover that either you don't like it as much as you thought you did or, a single forkful or bite is more than sufficient to undo the glamor spell they seem to hold over you.

Neither should I have to remind you that we are maintaining an average natural fast of at least 16 hours a day. Remember, we are interested in the *average!* Some days will naturally be longer, other days naturally shorter. Your brain-body seems to settle on averages. In the next chapter, when we talk about genetics and metabolism, we'll see this illustrated a bit more clearly. Changing the averages and sustaining the changes over a long enough period of time is how we create a new normal in our lives.

By now, you should also have begun to see increases in your energy, especially if you have been increasing your activity levels incrementally. To keep going, you'll have to make time for sustaining increased activities. You might consider taking up a local business's offer for free introductory lessons, as I mentioned before, or you can pick up something new. You can now see that small changes add up over time to big differences.

There are three aspects to successful long-term activity change. First, you must be moving. That much is obvious. The second is that you must enjoy the activity. If you don't enjoy it, you won't do it. That doesn't mean you don't have to work at getting better. That part is what makes the process engaging. And finally, for most people, a prosocial aspect to the activity is very motivating. Find things to do with others, even if it is as simple as walking your dog along a route where you see familiar faces. We are primarily social beings, and activities are one of the few ways we can actually make new friends as adults.

Therapeutic Fasting Patterns

In the last stage, we experienced one or two 24-hour fasts in a week's time, and you were free to choose the days. That is, of course, the first and easiest pattern. Technically, we might call it **Two Weekly OMADs**.

At the current stage, we begin to play with different kinds of therapeutic intermittent fasting patterns. I recommend working through the patterns in order the first time you do them, just to experience them all and to teach your mind that you can do them with confidence. Which you choose to practice over and over will be a matter of your preferences. I've known clients to express preference for each. Whatever works best for you. But don't just take the easy way out. Try all the patterns and see how they make you feel.

You will remain at this stage until you reach your goal. From this point forward, you should engage in one of the following therapeutic intermittent fasting patterns on a weekly basis. These are presented in order of difficulty and are delivered all at once in order to provide you with some variety.

Three Staggered OMADs

This pattern is different from Two Weekly OMADs in that it involves *three sequential days*. If your interim meals are very low in carbohydrates, you will likely be in ketosis during most of this pattern.

The staggering of the OMADs is easiest to understand if you are still eating three meals per day during an 8-hour eating window. On the first day, eat breakfast. After you finish your breakfast, eat nothing again until lunch the next day. Have a full meal that does not contain carbohydrates. Avoid them entirely, if possible, but all vegetables have some amount of carbohydrates. After you finish lunch, eat nothing again until dinner the following day. Your meal should not contain any carbohydrates at all. After you finish dinner, eat nothing again until dinner the next day. After you finish your dinner, do not eat again until after your natural fast has passed. Then eat as is your custom on non-fasting, natural fast days.

Participants who eat only two meals a day will go lunch to lunch, lunch to dinner, and dinner to dinner.

You will have noticed that the fasting pattern for two of the three days is a bit longer than 24 hours. You can do it! This pattern will help you prepare for the next.

The 36-Hour Fast

Begin the evening before your busiest day of the week. Finish eating at 7 p.m. or later. You already understand that if you were doing OMAD, you could eat any time after that hour the next day. This time, when your OMAD would be complete, you take only a glass of water, perhaps with a bit of lemon or lime, and/or a splash of raw apple cider vinegar. Go to bed early if you need to. You can eat any time after the hour you established the next morning. If it was 7 p.m., you can eat any time after 7 a.m.

In the 36-hour fast, you are taking advantage of two natural fasts, in which most of the time is spent sleeping. You don't have to eat at 7 a.m. You probably won't feel hungry at that time anyway. If your 36-hour fast becomes 40 hours because you wait until lunch, all the better.

You can easily make this fast a 48-hour fast by waiting until 7 p.m. It's easy if you keep busy. I'll discuss longer fasts later in this chapter, but for the purpose and under the instructions for this process, a 36-hour fast is the longest we will cover. You should do two 36-hour fasts during the week.

The Winning Hand

Surprisingly, this pattern is one of the most popular among my clients. Start with a 36-hour fast that ends at lunch or dinnertime. Have a well-portioned, no-carbohydrate meal, eating until you are satisfied. Then go into a 24-hour fast. After that, have another no-carbohydrate meal until you are satisfied. Follow that meal with another 36-hour fast.

Longer Fasts

I've already mentioned how easy it is to push a 36-hour fast to a 48-hour fast. My first 72-hour fast happened completely by accident, but I'm glad it did. I had planned a fast that ended with an evening meal. That day, I was held up at work and traffic was bad. I got home too late to eat. I suffered from acid reflux disease, and eating just before bed was always a recipe for a sleepless night, so I just went to bed. My 36-hour fast became 48.

I was no longer accustomed to eating breakfast. Eating at 7 or 8 a.m. just wasn't part of my circadian rhythm. I wasn't hungry, so I didn't eat. I forgot to bring food to work, so my next meal would have to be dinner. Forty-eight hours became sixty. I had a last-minute client, and again, I got home too late to eat. I went to bed and fell asleep while reading. Sometime the next day, I ate. Without planning it, I had fasted for more than 72 hours.

My longest fast at the time of this writing is five days. I did it because I wanted to see if I could and how it would feel. It felt great. For many people, the second fasting day is the most difficult. For me, the most difficult day is (and I expect it will always be) the first. Once I hit 24 hours, I'm good to go. At the end of my five-day fast, I considered making it seven days. It would have been easy. I decided against it. I don't remember why. The important thing is that I know that I can fast for an amount of time most people consider inconceivable. So can you.

The main advantage of longer fasts is increased autophagy, where the body literally consumes weak and redundant material to create its own fuel. It's a kind of cleansing process that has terrific benefits for healing when diseases, like cancer, depend on blood glucose levels. Once the body reaches a certain degree of ketosis, ketones (not glucose) are the primary sources of energy. Those glucose hungry diseases starve.

Helpful Fasting Reminders

- **Stay hydrated** and get enough salt. Drink plenty of filtered water. You can use a small wedge of lemon or lime to make it a bit more exciting.

- **Plan the next meal** that will break your fast. Plan what you will eat and when. You can always change your mind. Remember to use self-suggestion. Phrase your plan as, "I will eat _____ sometime after _____ o'clock.

- **Stay busy and keep your mind occupied.** Choose busy days or make them busy. Feel free to exercise or work out if that is your preference.

- **Monitor your internal monologue** and if you catch yourself sinking into negativity, intentionally make your monologue more positive

- **Acknowledge, observe, and unpack feelings of hunger** but identify the source and the trigger. You might be legitimately hungry but use self-suggestion to remind your brain-body what you are doing and why.

- **Acknowledge, observe and unpack cravings.** Remember that cravings are a distraction. Cravings are usually purposeful, seeking to distract you from something even slightly unpleasant. Take time to address and confront whatever is bothering you. Fasting can heal the heart, the mind as well as the body.

- **Drink as much as you want.** Water, black unsweetened coffee or tea, herbal teas hot or cold.

- **Take your medications.** Take all your normal medications but be careful about hypoglycemia if you are still taking any diabetes medication capable of causing low blood sugar. If medications suggest being taken with food, this is usually to avoid stomach upset but know for sure. Sometimes, it is to facilitate absorption. If you need to eat something with your medications, consider a few olives, nuts, or a small piece of cheese. These will technically break your fast but not for long. They might extend feelings of hunger.

- **Prepare your escape plan,** if necessary. (Chapter Eleven)

- **Use ketone test strips** to gauge when you enter ketosis and to what degree of ketosis you experience at the end of the fast.

- **Don't weigh yourself** as any weight you lose

during an extended fast will almost surely come back. Intermittent fasting is intermittent to avoid sending the body into prolonged starvation mode.

- **Avoid carbohydrates in the meal that breaks your fast.**

Remember that we are not fasting to avoid calories. Fasting is caloric deprivation, but for the purpose of allowing the body to engage in activities and functions it may have rarely used in the past. Just like when we exercise, we are burning glucose, not calories. When we fast, we encourage ketosis and increase autophagy. That's what makes therapeutic intermittent fasting therapeutic.

body's idle.

You burn energy when you are sitting quietly, doing nothing. You even burn energy when you are asleep. If you believe you have a slow metabolism, you may be right; particularly if you have chronically dieted, followed reduced-calorie diets, or temporarily followed any restrictive diet.

Permanent success depends on establishing a new normal for your body. This requires an adjustment to your metabolism.

Before I go any farther, I want you to avoid supplements that promise an increased metabolism as they may contain ephedrine-like stimulants. Shun energy drinks, which are usually loaded with caffeine and sugar. Avoid over-the-counter diet pills or supplements. They are a waste of your money, and you need to stop screwing around with your system. If your doctor has prescribed a diet pill, take time to actually read what the medication is, what it does, and what the side effects might be. By now, you are taking more ownership and responsibility for your wellness and information about medications, interactions, and side effects are readily available online.

The best way to effect a change in your metabolism is to eat a healthy, well-balanced diet and to gradually increase your activity level to effectively use the fuel and nutrition you consume.

become natural—that is, normal—for you.

Most of us do not know what it means to eat sufficient quantities of nutrient-dense food. Most of what we have consumed over the years has been nutrient sparse or artificially enriched with chemical nutrients we might not even be able to absorb.

Nutrition is not easy because, as a society, we do not eat the kind of food that naturally provides it. Start eating the food your body thrives on, and you will eventually crave that, and not the junk.

There are some nutrients that are commonly lacking in our cultural diet. If you think you need a supplement, you should know why you need it and why you are not getting it from your food. Learn how to naturally acquire that nutrient in your diet.

Activity and Metabolism

If you park your car in the garage and do not touch it for three months, you may have a bit of difficulty starting it when you need it. Some folks are amazed that their bodies creak, that they have pain, stiffness, and weakness when they sit on their butts all day. It is convenient to blame it on getting older, but it is really just our sedentary lifestyle.

How long can you stand up without wanting to sit down? How far can you walk without wanting to take a breather? How much physical work can you do without feeling stiff or achy the next day?

If finding a fun movement has to this point eluded you, start somewhere. Anywhere. Do not set artificial goals that you can't sustain. Keep going with more steps tomorrow than today until you find something. It will happen. Consider learning how to stretch correctly for flexibility. Walk more and stretch. Combine a stretching sequence with relaxing, focused self-hypnosis and you'll not only tone your body, but you'll also reduce stress and anxiety.

Your posture, walking, and increasing your flexibility are good places to start. They may not be enjoyable at first, but they can lead to finding an amazing activity that you love. When you are ready to explore, if you haven't done so already, consider taking advantage of free classes in your area.

Classes are great because they are prosocial. That means we are more motivated to attend, more motivated to improve, and we benefit from sharing an experience with other people. There are lots of group classes available, and many will offer you a free session to see if you would like to attend. You will get a sales pitch after. Just do not sign up if you are not sure; and if you do, sign up only for a minimum number of classes to make sure you really like it. I have had clients who have tried yoga, Zumba, Tai Chi, belly dancing, and even pole dancing. There are dance classes in tap, ballroom, and salsa. Almost all martial arts classes seem to offer a free class or two to the curious.

Remember, real sustainable activity is about enjoyment and getting good at something. It is not about routine exercise, burning calories, or necessarily building muscle.

Hire a personal trainer for a minimum number of sessions. The trainer should discuss your goals, any limiting conditions, and then guide you through a session that might leave you a little sore the next day but feeling good about yourself.

If you do not want to drop money on something like that, there are many things you can do on your own, using instructional videos that are actually free on YouTube. You want to be careful and proceed slowly because doing exercises the wrong way can actually cause physical damage.

Whatever you explore and finally choose, you will probably be pretty bad at it at first. Ask yourself, "Would I enjoy getting good at this?" Notice I did not say, "being good at this." You have to enjoy getting good at it. That often means working hard at it.

While the movement is important, enjoyment is critical. You will discover that that activity is part of you. If you have a body, it needs to move. The phrase "use it or lose it" has never been truer. There is a condition called "learned non-use." It means that we learn to not use certain parts of our body and allow other parts to attempt to do the job.

As your regular and consistent activity levels rise, your metabolism adjusts to accommodate the energy costs of the movement.

Your Metabolic Mind

We often don't consider the mental and emotional factors

that have a strong influence on metabolism, but the relationship is obvious. We know, for example, that physical exercise can reduce depression. While we know about emotional eating, there is a more subtle relationship among emotions, attitudes, and even thoughts that impact brain-body function.

We know, for example, that stress releases cortisol, which can cause us to resist weight loss and may even cause us to gain weight. There are both physical and mental kinds of stress, making the attitudes we hold able to impact metabolism either indirectly or directly.

Many people have experienced success with hypnosis for weight loss, even when it is still considered a matter of overeating and self-control. In fact, I know a lot of hypnotists whose sessions focus on portion control hypnosis and aversion therapy, such as making chocolate taste like liver and onions. Sometimes it works, if only for a while.

Hypnosis works on automatic thoughts, reactions, feelings, and behaviors, all of which factor into metabolism. These things drive how we feel, and how we feel drives hormonal reactions in the body. Those hormonal reactions can have a strong effect on metabolism, the immune system, our motivations, and our confidence.

Your internal monologue or narrative is a form of self-hypnosis. In effect, you are telling yourself a story that makes or affirms self-hypnotic suggestions to your unconscious mind. You can utilize self-hypnosis by recognizing counterproductive thoughts and correcting them, making them productive in the way you want them to be. You are thus making self-hypnotic suggestions. Gradually, that new story becomes true for you.

Hypnotically, if we think or nurture the attitude that we are starving, our bodies may respond by going into starvation mode even when we have plenty to eat. Your internal monologue, or the way you narrate your life, is critical. When you tell yourself you cannot eat something, all you think about is eating that thing, and you feel the loss or absence of that food. You automatically and unconsciously set up a goal to eat that food again as soon as you can, and often as much as you can.

Healthy eating attitudes and balanced eating emotions can go a long way toward convincing your body to freely use the resources available to it, including that stored fat that it had been saving for lean times. Remember that from now on, we are choosing to eat intentionally.

In traditional weight loss hypnosis, some hypnotists call that process of letting go of the fat "releasing" the fat. It is often accomplished through regression hypnosis, in which a client may reexperience an event, condition, or circumstance through unconscious memory. If your body is holding onto fat, there may well be an unrecognized sense of insecurity. Once the insecurity is gone, the body will freely use that fat as a fuel source.

I had a friend who began working as a teller at a bank. One customer, an elderly homeless woman who carried with her a very unpleasant odor, would come into the bank to withdraw tiny amounts of cash, five dollars or less. No one wanted to take care of her because of her odor, and the other tellers thought it humorous to direct her to my friend's window. When he looked up her account, she had enough money to comfortably live for years—perhaps the rest of her life—in an apartment of her own.

The body might well be refusing to utilize its fat reserves because of unconscious or emotional insecurity. It sounds fantastic, but I've seen phenomena as a hypnotist, though I can only provide anecdotal evidence. The man who wanted to lose weight but unconsciously enjoyed the imposing, even intimidating figure his size afforded him. The woman, a high-powered corporate executive, who said she believed her weight held back her career but suffered from imposter syndrome, not believing she was qualified or living up to the status and position she had achieved. One man believed he was single because his approaches were rejected by prospective dates. He liked to assume the rejections were due to his weight. Later, it came out that if he lost weight and was still single, the rejection would be more personal.

I'm not a psychotherapist, I'm a hypnotist. Things like this come out in client sessions, sometimes when progress in terms of weight is elusive. These unhealthy thought patterns, be they conscious or unconscious, can underlie the reasons for emotional eating, binge eating, and even eating disorders. If I think there might be a legitimate eating disorder, I refer the client to someone qualified to make the diagnosis. Of course, I am more than willing to collaborate with that mental health professional.

Chapter Fifteen: The Home Stretch

If you have not already reached your goal, you should be well on your way. Just keep going and learning as much as you can about your body. And remember the following key principles:

Eat mindfully and intentionally. Casual snacking or grazing is a thing of the past. We do not live to eat. We eat to live. Eating mindfully and intentionally helps our brain-body learn when to initiate cephalic digestive responses.

Nurture the mind-body relationship. Keep your attitudes and habits synchronized for health. Resist reverting to old thought patterns and habits. Most people who go on a diet think when they reach their goal, the diet ends. Our plan, on the other hand, is a comfortable life-long process of managing wellness.

Keep indulgences in perspective. Rare Indulgence is a thing for celebrations, not a reward for doing well or compensation for a difficult time.

Keep mixing up your eating and fasting patterns so that your brain-body does not settle into a new normal until you are ready. If your progress slows down or you reach a plateau (a time when you seem to be in a holding pattern and not making progress), do something to shake things up. You can reduce your natural fast for a few days and then do a series of staggered OMADs. You might choose to do a fast longer than you ever have. You might stagger your movement and activities. Or you might take a short vacation, relax, and have some fun.

As you approach your goal, it is time to reconsider how you imagine forever—your new normal—to look. You will not be imagining the life you might have when you first started this process. What sorts of foods will remain a part of your regular diet? Will you want to go keto, or will you want to incorporate a bit more carbohydrates? What about the role of sugar in your life? What average natural fast will you maintain?

Keep in mind that while easing off of the strict rules may be part of your decision, any one of them can limit your ultimate success or lead to sliding back into old patterns.

I titled the book of my own diabetes reversal, *Deleting Diabetes*, as a nod to the notion that when we delete a file from our computer, it doesn't disappear from the hard drive but is only ignored. The file remains intact until it has been overwritten. A forensic data professional can easily locate and open a file that remains on a hard drive. Given the size of hard drives today, I wonder if any files ever get overwritten.

My diabetes has been deleted. My new normal is pretty stable, and I really do have more wiggle room in my diet than I did when I was actively in the program. To date, I am still not diabetic, but there is an inkling in the back of my mind that the file still exists and that it would be easy for me to recover it and restore it.

For this reason, I still maintain a decent and comfortable natural fast and occasionally, once every three to six weeks, choose to engage in therapeutic intermittent fasting, something I will do for the rest of my life. I may not do it as often as I once did, but I keep in practice and often test to see how deeply into ketosis I am.

On that score, I think I am in and out of ketosis depending on what I have eaten. I know that if I do a 24-hour fast, I am in some measurable degree of ketosis. In my mind, that means that my body continues to use up glycogen stores in a reasonable amount of time.

When you reach your goal, continue monitoring your changes and remain conscious of your brain-body. Eat nutritious food, stay active, and thrive in life. You may choose to adjust your efforts but live according to your new normal. Make every attempt to stabilize at that level for at least a year. To a certain degree, your new normal lifestyle is and will continue to be important for the rest of your life. May it be ever more abundant.

Joseph A. Onesta

Recommended Reading

I consider the following books essential reading. Amazingly, they are all old enough to find in a used bookstore, and all of them are available in audio versions.

Ken Berry, M.D, *Lies My Doctor Told Me*

Jason Fung, M.D, *The Cancer Code*

Jason Fung, M.D, *The Diabetes Code*

Jason Fung, M.D., The Obesity Code

Lierre Keith, *The Vegetarian Myth (a little heavy handed but still worth it.)*

Tim Noakes and Marika Sboros, *Real Food on Trial*

David Perlmutter and Kristin Loberg, *Brain Maker*

David Perlmutter and Kristin Loberg, *Grain Brain*

Gary Taubes, Good Calories, *Bad Calories*

Gary Taubes, *Why We Get Fat*

Nina Teicholz, *The Big Fat Surprise*

Joseph A. Onesta

About the Author

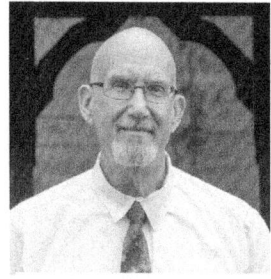

Joseph A. Onesta is an author and clinical hypnosis practitioner in Pittsburgh, Pennsylvania. He works with clients in person in his practice, Mind Power Pittsburgh. He also works with clients from around the world online.

Joseph is a frequent speaker at international hypnosis conferences, and as a certified hypnosis instructor, he supervises the practice of a small number of new hypnosis practitioners. He is a dynamic public speaker and provides speaker services to organizations.

His other books are, in order of publication: *The Hypnofasting Program Guide: A Practical Plan to Lose Weight and Control Type 2 Diabetes*; *Uneasy Faith: How to Survive Religious Trauma without Sacrificing Spirituality*; *Deleting Diabetes: I Did It. You Can, Too*; *Life Without Diabetes: Manage And Reverse Type 2 Diabetes in Weeks Without Starving or Counting Calories;* and *The Hypnotist's Guide to Diabetes and Obesity*.

Joseph lives in Pittsburgh, Pennsylvania with his husband Elihu and their finicky cat, Abbey. He may be contacted through his company website, www.mindpowerpittsburgh.com or www.josephonesta.com

Made in the USA
Middletown, DE
25 May 2024